## Benefits and Risks of Hormone Replacement Therapy (HRT)

The decision whether to take hormone replacement therapy (HRT) is one that each woman must make for herself, in consultation with her primary care physician and gynecologist. There are many factors to consider, without one being more important than the others. Here is a summary of the general benefits and risks of HRT, as we currently understand them.

**Benefits of HRT:**

➤ HRT relieves many of the discomforts of menopause, including hot flashes, mood swings, irregular bleeding, and vaginal dryness.

➤ HRT protects your bones from calcium and mineral loss, helping to prevent or delay osteoporosis.

➤ HRT lowers blood lipid levels, which may reduce the risk of heart disease and stroke.

➤ HRT affects neurotransmitters in the brain, helping to improve memory and cognitive functions.

➤ HRT may prevent or delay Alzheimer's disease.

**Risks of HRT:**

➤ HRT can increase the risk for developing breast cancer, particularly in women who already face a higher risk than normal.

➤ Estrogen-only HRT (without progesterone) increases the risk for endometrial cancer in women who still have their uteruses.

➤ HRT can result in periodlike bleeding that continues for six months to a year.

➤ HRT can cause side effects such as migraine headaches, fluid retention, weight gain, breast tenderness, and PMS-like symptoms.

➤ Progesterone replacement can cause or worsen mood swings and depression.

# Integrative Approaches to Managing Menopause

Numerous complementary therapies can make the menopause journey more pleasant. Most have only short-term effects and don't provide the protection against heart disease and osteoporosis that HRT does. Here is a summary of integrative therapies for menopause; discuss these therapies with your primary care physician or gynecologist to determine what's right to help ease your menopause passage to wise womanhood.

| Complementary Therapy | Beneficial Effects | Risks |
| --- | --- | --- |
| Acupuncture | Relieves many of the discomforts of menopause, including hot flashes | None, if practitioner is qualified and uses sterile, disposable needles |
| Biofeedback | Relieves stress, hot flashes, headaches | None |
| Herbal remedies | Estrogenlike substances may relieve discomforts such as hot flashes, mood swings, and vaginal dryness | Some herbal products can interact with each other or other medications |
| Massage | Relieves stress and general feelings of discomfort | None |
| Meditation | Relieves stress, hot flashes, headaches, and general discomforts | None |
| Phytoestrogens | Soy isoflavones are especially effective for hot flashes, mood swings, and vaginal dryness | Some women may not like the taste of soy-based foods; might not give long-term protection from key health risks, although studies are ongoing and promising |
| Yoga | Stretches and tones skeletal structures; relieves stress | Slight risk of injury |

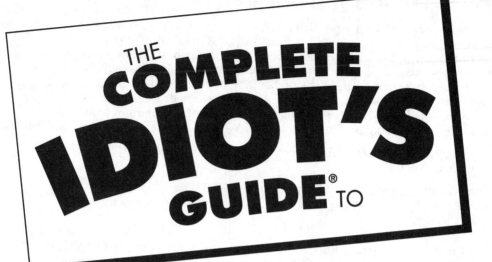

# Menopause

by Maureen Miller Pelletier, M.D.,
and Deborah S. Romaine

**alpha books**

Macmillan USA, Inc.
201 West 103rd Street
Indianapolis, IN 46290

A Pearson Education Company

*$ 2.—*

**Publisher**
*Marie Butler-Knight*

**Product Manager**
*Phil Kitchel*

**Managing Editor**
*Cari Luna*

**Acquisitions Editors**
*Mike Sanders*
*Susan Zingraf*

**Book Producer**
*Lee Ann Chearney/Amaranth*

**Development Editor**
*Lynn Northrup*

**Production Editor**
*JoAnna Kremer*

**Copy Editor**
*Krista Hansing*

**Cartoonist**
*Jody P. Schaeffer*

**Cover Designers**
*Mike Freeland*
*Kevin Spear*

**Book Designers**
*Scott Cook and Amy Adams of DesignLab*

**Indexer**
*Angie Bess*

**Layout/Proofreading**
*Svetlana Dominguez*
*Ayanna Lacey*

# Contents at a Glance

# Contents

## 7   Do You Need Your Uterus? Hysterectomies and Surgical Menopause      65

## 8   Early Menopause      77

# Foreword

When I was first asked to write a foreword for a book whose title started with *The Complete Idiot's Guide to …* I was highly skeptical. I assumed that it would be a mockery of menopause, a take-off on self-help books. Yet out of curiosity, I agreed to look over the pages. Imagine my surprise when I indeed read the book and discovered a wonderful combination of up-to-date medical information, compassionate advice, and humor. And to my chagrin, I actually learned a lot (which at some level makes the title even harder to take!).

According to the media, menopause is "huge." Millions of baby boomers are going through this transition every year, and this segment of population is well-known for educating themselves and taking action to improve their health. Dozens of books on menopause come out annually, but most have not done well. There are a number of reasons for this: Some books are too medical, many focus on the hormone-replacement debate but only argue either pro or con, some are written by menopause "survivors" and can make the process sound unbearable, and many are simply boring!

*The Complete Idiot's Guide to Menopause* is different. Although co-authored by a physician, the medical information is clear and easily understood. There is information presented on both the pros and cons of hormone replacement therapy (HRT), which will allow the reader, in collaboration with her own physician, to make the decision from an informed, careful perspective. There is a plethora of advice on alternatives to HRT, ranging from lifestyle changes to herbs. The book is written with a reassuring tone, and readers will come away with the impression that menopause is a natural process that requires some adaptation but that it should in no way feel overwhelming. As a scientist, I loved the fact that the book was medically accurate, with no New Age unresearched promises. As a woman, I loved the humor, the approach, and the empathy.

The potential reader may wonder why it is important to be educated about menopause. After all, it is a natural process that all women will go through. There are a number of reasons why it is vital for women to understand the medical and psychological impact of menopause. First of all, a woman's risk of certain diseases, such as heart disease, rises sharply after menopause. In order to maintain or achieve maximum health, she will need to pay attention to her lifestyle habits and may need to make modifications that were not as necessary prior to menopause. Although women fear breast cancer more than heart disease, heart disease poses a far greater risk to our health. Second, the biological changes that occur during menopause may have an impact on our psychological health. Symptoms of depression, anger, and anxiety may increase during the menopausal years. Contrary to popular belief, merely going through "the change" does not make one become a raving bitchy lunatic. However, having hot flashes at night can lead to chronic sleep deprivation, which in turn can lead to depression. Learning how to decrease hot flashes at night, either through HRT or by changing your diet and sleeping habits, can solve the problem.

One of the many strengths of this book is the inclusion and responsible description of complementary and alternative approaches. As the debate on the pros and cons of HRT increases in the medical community (does HRT increase the risk of breast cancer? can HRT reduce or increase the risk of heart disease? is HRT the best way to prevent the development of osteoporosis?), many women are turning to other approaches, some of which have been proven to relieve certain menopausal symptoms, and some of which may harm them. Up-to-date information on these approaches is included, with appropriate cautions for the approaches that warrant them.

You will enjoy reading this book. You will learn, you will be forced to think, and you will laugh. And most of all, you will become healthier.

Have fun.


Alice D. Domar, Ph.D.

Alice D. Domar, Ph.D., directs the Mind/Body Center for Women's Health at the Mind/Body Medical Institute, Beth Israel Deaconess Medical Center, and Harvard Medical School. She is the author of *Healing Mind, Healthy Woman* (Dell, 1997), *Self-Nurture* (Viking, 2000), and *The Harvard Medical School Fertility Program* (Simon & Schuster, 2000). Dr. Domar's accomplishments have earned her a national and international reputation as a leading women's health expert, and she has appeared on *Good Morning America, ABC News, Dateline NBC,* and *The Today Show,* as well as in numerous print publications.

# Introduction

How do you feel about your impending menopause? Are you excited about traveling the next transition of your life, or apprehensive about the changes your journey might bring? Many women vacillate between the two poles, not certain where to stand. But there is a middle ground—and we present it here, in *The Complete Idiot's Guide to Menopause*.

Menopause is both a unique and universal journey for all women who travel its path. Because it's universal, we know a lot about what happens within your body and your mind. Because it's unique, your menopause experience won't be quite the same as anyone else's. This guide gives you the foundation of knowledge that you need to travel your journey of transformation with confidence and anticipation.

## How to Use This Book

This book is organized into seven parts:

**Part 1, "Enter Prime Time,"** introduces the history and mythology of menopause.

**Part 2, "Midlife Metamorphosis,"** presents preparations that take place in your body and mind to get ready for menopause.

**Part 3, "Ch-Ch-Changes: Menopause Symptoms,"** features the changes—physical, emotional, and spiritual—that take place during menopause.

**Part 4, "HRT or No HRT, That Is the Question,"** discusses the various medical treatments available for menopause discomforts as well as to help prevent future health problems.

**Part 5, "Menopause Treatment *Au Naturel*,"** takes a look at the remedies from Mother Nature.

**Part 6, "Self-Care While You're Going Through Menopause,"** shows you how to draw upon the experience and wisdom of the ages to shape and guide your menopause journey.

**Part 7, "Vibrant, Feminine, Wise, and Wonderful,"** tells you how to take care of your body after menopause so that it will continue taking care of you for the rest of your long, healthy life.

# Tips and Tidbits

In each chapter, we've included boxes that present interesting and helpful information.

**Wise Up**

These boxes describe and explain technical terms.

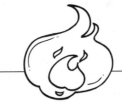

**Hot Flash!**

These boxes give warnings and cautions.

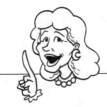

**Wise Woman's Wisdom**

These boxes feature quotes from famous—and not so famous—women who have something to say about being a woman.

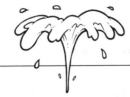

**Wellspring**

These boxes present interesting and informative tidbits and factoids about menopause and related topics.

**Embracing Change**

These boxes give helpful hints and suggestions.

# Acknowledgments

It takes a team to write a book, and we give thanks to the wonderful people who've brought this book to life. In particular, we thank the team at Alpha Books, including publisher Marie Butler-Knight, acquistions editors Mike Sanders and Susan Zingraf, development editor Lynn Northrup, and production editor JoAnna Kremer.

Debbie gives special thanks to the women of the Narrows Glen writer's group, octogenarians and nonagenarians all, who are joyous evidence that the wise woman thrives. She also thanks Mike, Chris, and Cass for their patience and support; Ava for her unwavering friendship; and Lee Ann Chearney at Amaranth for the wisdom of her guidance.

Maureen especially thanks her mom, Rachel Cote Miller, for always telling her that there is no such word as "can't"; her husband of 28 years, Roger, who has always provided endless support for her and their daughters and who gives her a little healthy prodding by saying "go for it!" Maureen also thanks her daughters Nicole and Monique who assure her that she's a "super mom" but would like to see her more—to the point of coming to her hospital call room overnight to be with her; and Sandy Arnold, her medical assistant, who is with her more than anybody else and who puts up with her quirkiness and demands.

## *Special Thanks to the Technical Editor*

*The Complete Idiot's Guide to Menopause* was reviewed by an expert who not only checked the accuracy of what you'll learn in this book, but also provided invaluable insight to help ensure that this book tells you everything you need to know about menopause. Our special thanks are extended to Mary Eileen Buban, Psy.D.

Mary Eileen Buban, Psy.D., is a clinical psychologist in private practice in Cincinnati, Ohio. Dr. Buban's current interests and projects include women's health issues, disaster/trauma response services, psychological services to private and charter schools, and medical expert work with the Social Security Administration. She is interested in integrative healing methods and has received training in Reiki and Energy Psychology. Dr. Buban and Maureen Miller Pelletier, M.D., have designed Integrative Treatment for Chronic Pelvic Pain Groups, and are committed to providing women with the knowledge and tools to enhance their healthcare needs.

# Trademarks

All terms mentioned in this book that are known to be or are suspected of being trademarks or service marks have been appropriately capitalized. Alpha Books and Macmillan USA, Inc., cannot attest to the accuracy of this information. Use of a term in this book should not be regarded as affecting the validity of any trademark or service mark.

# Part 1

# Enter Prime Time

*Just when your life is tracking the way you want it to, Mother Nature shows up with other plans. It's menopause, and it's about to become the path that will lead you through the rest of your life. As much as this is your personal journey, it's also the odyssey of women since the beginning of time.*

*One important factor sets you apart from those who have traveled this path before you: Yours is the first generation for which menopause is truly a marker of midlife, not the alarm of impending demise. You can expect 30, 40, 50, or more years of enjoyable living. So read on, and prepare to cross the threshold to the rest of your life!*

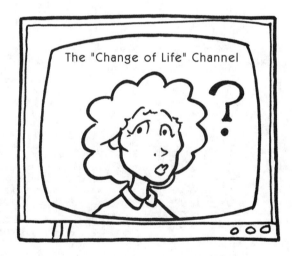

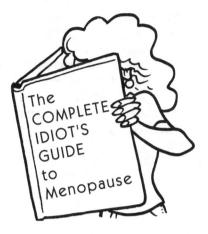

# What Is Menopause?

In the year 2000, nearly 52 million American women were age 45 or older. Two million of them will enter menopause each year for the next 20 years. For the first time in history, a woman can expect to spend as much or more of her life after her child-bearing years as she did during them. This is shifting our perception of what it means to be in the "prime" of life.

Medical technology is further shifting perceptions, establishing an environment (in our Western culture) in which menopause has become a "medical condition" for doctors to monitor, treat, and control. This has advantages and disadvantages. Medications and other therapies can relieve many of menopause's discomforts. But the view that menopause needs medical intervention can cause discomforts of another sort for women who want to guide themselves through their menopause journeys.

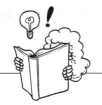

# Navigating the Silent Passage

Women have passed through the life transition known as *menopause* since the beginning of time. There is nothing new about this. Menopause is a natural and normal stage in the cycle of life that defines a woman. Until recently, however, women have made this passage secretly and in silence, as though it were somehow unnatural or dangerous. Women going through "the change"—our grandmothers and even our mothers—were expected to keep any signs of it to themselves. Unbelievably, the word *menopause* didn't appear in the title of an American book until the 1980s.

A lot has changed since then. Much has been written about the phenomenal influence of the generation known as the Baby Boomers—those born between the mid-1940s and the late 1950s. They are the largest generation to sweep through population demographics in the history of the United States. The women among them have redefined what it means to be a woman in today's world. They have redefined career and family, and they are redefining menopause.

## A Woman's Life Is a Circle

From ancient times, we have perceived the environment in which we live as a collection of cycles, circles of events that take place on certain schedules. There is the cycle of the day, marked by alternating periods of light and darkness as the Earth rotates on its axis (an imaginary line between the North and South Poles). There is the cycle of the month, marked by the phases of the moon as it revolves around the Earth. There is the cycle of the year, marked by the changing seasons as the Earth completes its orbit around the sun.

We have used—and still use—these patterns to define the passage of time. Sunrise defines the start of each new day. The brightness of the full moon denotes the completion of a month (though this doesn't correspond to our 12-month calendar because a lunar month is 29.5 days long and our calendar months range from 28 to 31 days in length). And the changing of the seasons defines the cycle of life.

### Of Cycles: Menstrual and Life

Early cultures perceived a woman's menstrual cycle to follow the cycle of the moon. The Greek philosopher Aristotle (384–322 B.C.E.) was among the first to record this observation in writing. He was a little too precise, however, asserting that every woman menstruated at the same time each month. Of course, this is not true, although some studies have observed that women who live together for long periods, such as college roommates, tend to find that their cycles coincide over time.

Many people believe that the cycles of life are linked to one another or are smaller or larger representations of each other. In this view, the monthly menstrual cycle is a shadow of the yearly cycle of seasons. Each quarter of the menstrual cycle correlates to a season of the year: ovulation and spring, the week following ovulation and summer, menstruation and autumn, and the week following menstruation and winter. By the same token, a woman's life correlates to the seasons of the year: the spring of her youth, the summer of her fertility, the autumn of her childrearing, and the winter of her menopause. After menopause comes the second spring—a rebirth into a new life.

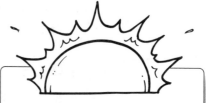

**Embracing Change**

Menopause itself is not associated with any immediate increased risk of health problems. The overall risk of conditions such as heart disease and osteoporosis naturally increases with age, in men as well as in women. Women can do much to offset their risks by making lifestyle habits such as good nutrition and regular exercise part of their daily lives.

## Luna: Maiden, Enchantress, Mother, Wise Woman

The moon affects many Earth cycles. It draws the tides of the oceans in and out. Farmers have long planted by the new moon and harvested by the full moon, a cycle that synchronizes nicely with the seasons of nature. In mythology, the moon has been a symbol of the feminine since ancient times. Given *yin*, or feminine, attributes by ancient astrologers, the moon represents fertility and motherhood. Kuan-yin, the Japanese goddess of motherhood, bestows the gift of children upon desiring couples. The Roman goddess Luna (also known as Artemis) danced in the light of the moon, bringing fertility to those who joined her. As the mother image in mythology, the moon both nurtures and protects.

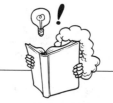

**Wise Up**

**Yin** and its counterpart **yang** represent the duality, or two coexisting elements, of life energy. Yin is the feminine energy—passive, receptive, cool, shady or dark, and wet. Yang is the masculine energy—active, giving, warm, light, and dry.

The moon was believed to have other less positive influences as well. While ancient Greek physicians believed that moonlight could cure warts, they also cautioned against trimming corns or cutting hair while the moon was full. Ancient physicians in several cultures believed that the moon caused erratic behavior—hence the term *lunatic* for the insane, who were believed to be *moonstruck*. Medical texts from the twelfth century warned of the dangers of sleeping in the moonlight or letting the light of the moon shine through the bedchamber's window to touch those sleeping within. This, said the texts, was certain to cause lunacy.

It didn't take long for people to link a woman's body cycles with the cycles of the moon, with understandably mixed connotations given the confused beliefs about the moon's influences. Some ancient cultures revered a woman's monthly cycles, connecting them with fertility and new life. Others feared them, interpreting menstrual bleeding as the body's attempt to rid itself of unpleasantness or even poisons.

Of course, we know now that a woman's menstrual cycle signals fertility for her, not for the season's crops. We know that menstrual bleeding is a natural and healthful part of fertility, as the uterus sheds its lining, not toxins, in preparation for the next month's cycle. And we know that moonlight has nothing to do with lunacy, erratic behavior, warts, corns, or bad hair days.

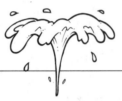

### Wellspring

We owe our concept of a seven-day week to the ancient Egyptians, who believed that there were seven planets orbiting the Earth and named one day for each of them. We now know, of course, that the moon is the only astral body that orbits the Earth, which is itself a planet and not the axis of the universe. By the fourth century, the Romans had adopted this system and spread it throughout Europe. A century later, the Anglo-Saxons translated *lunae dies*, "the day of the moon," into Old English as *monandaeg*—what we know today as Monday. Monday's child may be fair of face, as the children's poem goes, but she is also Luna's daughter.

# The Climacteric Stage: We're Not Talking About the Weather

The *climacteric*—sounds like it's time to run for cover! But the climacteric is not a weather situation. From the same Greek root word as *climax*, climacteric means "peak" or "culmination." A climacteric is a significant turning point in a sequence of events. In botany, climacteric refers to the rapid rise in the carbon dioxide/oxygen exchange in plants just before fruit reaches full ripeness. In the human life cycle, climacteric is another term for menopause.

In some respects, climacteric is perhaps a better term than menopause to define this transition in a woman's life because it implies continuation in an ongoing cycle. A climacteric is a major—but nonetheless single—step in a series of events that continues beyond it. Menopause is the time in a woman's life when she stops menstruating, yes, but her life cycle continues.

Many cultures view menopause more as a transition in the cycle of life, as the term *climacteric* implies, than as a defined state of health. In these cultures, women report far fewer "symptoms" than do American women. Fewer than 20 percent of Japanese women experience hot flashes, for example, while nearly half of American women do. This is not to suggest that the indications of menopause are all in your head. Your body is undergoing the most dramatic long-term changes it has experienced since puberty. These signs—hot flashes, mood swings, vaginal dryness—are very real and very physical.

What cultural differences in responding to menopause do suggest is that there are many ways to manage the signs. Viewing something as a normal aspect of a process has a great deal to do with what you perceive and how you react. Numerous studies have proven, for example, that surgery patients who know they will feel pain for a period of time after their operations recover more quickly and with less reported pain than those who have no idea what to expect. Likewise, women who know that menopause is a natural life transition through which they will pass—and come out at the other side—are less likely to view it as something that needs to be fixed.

**Wise Up**

**Climacteric** means a significant turning point or critical phase in a sequence of events. It comes from the Greek root that means "rung of a ladder." It is a word sometimes used to refer to menopause.

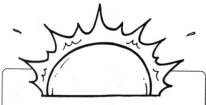

**Embracing Change**

About 80 percent of women experience only mild or occasional signs of the changes taking place during menopause. For many of them, menopause represents a transition to a new phase of their lives, a sort of rebirth or second spring.

## When Does Menopause Start?

Menopause starts when a woman's ovaries stop producing ripened eggs and her estrogen levels begin to decline. For most women, this happens sometime between age 50

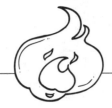

**Hot Flash!**

You can *still* become pregnant *during* menopause, even if you go several months between periods. You remain fertile until you've gone 12 consecutive months without a period.

and age 55, though natural menopause can begin when a woman is in her early 40s or not until she is near 60 (although there is a condition called premature ovarian failure that causes a woman to enter menopause well before her 40s).

Contrary to popular belief, there is no correlation between the age when you first started your period (called *menarche* in medical lingo) and the age when you enter menopause. Also contrary to popular belief, women are not entering menopause at a younger age than did women of previous generations. Although women today are starting their periods at an earlier age (around age 13, compared to around age 17 in 1900), they still enter menopause at about the same age as women have for centuries.

Researchers are still unclear about what role heredity might play in when a woman enters menopause. For many years, doctors believed that a woman whose mother and maternal grandmother entered menopause early would likely do the same—or vice versa, if your mother and your mother's mother entered menopause late in life. A number of studies have failed to support this correlation, however. Nor does there seem to be any connection between the timing of menopause and the number of pregnancies you've had or how long your monthly periods last. One lifestyle or environmental factor that does influence when you'll start menopause is cigarette smoking. Women who smoke enter menopause one to two years earlier than women who do not smoke. Researchers aren't sure why this is, although they suspect that nicotine, the major addictive chemical in tobacco, interferes with the ovary's ability to produce ripened eggs.

**Wise Up**

**Perimenopause** is the period of time when a woman's body is preparing for menopause. *Peri* means "before" or "around." Perimenopause can precede menopause by one or two to five or six years.

## How Long Does Menopause Last?

Menopause lasts two to three years for most women. Your passage through menopause is not complete until you've gone without menstrual periods for a full year. Most women experience a year or two of irregular periods and other indications that their bodies are beginning to change. Some women experience indications that menopause is on its way for as long as five or six years before they actually enter menopause. We now recognize this as a transition separate from menopause, which doctors have termed *perimenopause*. We discuss this in Chapter 4, "Perimenopause: Approaching Menopause."

## *Is There Life After Menopause?*

Until well into the twentieth century, doctors and women alike viewed menopause as the end of a woman's womanliness, as well as the beginning of the end of her life. With her ability to bear children gone, a woman was nothing but a shell without use or purpose in society. This was an easy conclusion to reach because women tended to enter menopause in their early 50s and died by their early 60s. Although we know now that menopause does nothing to usher in the end of life, neither women nor doctors knew that then. Little wonder that they feared and dreaded menopause!

Yes, indeed, there is life after menopause. For many women, it's a more confident and creative life. Most women find that menopause brings a sense of freedom into their lives unlike anything they've experienced as adults. No longer is unintended pregnancy a concern. For many women, menopause coincides with children leaving home as young adults to start their own lives. Most women are well established in their careers or are nearing retirement and considering other options.

# The Medicalization of Menopause

In the middle of the twentieth century, the art of medicine finally came into its own as a science. New discoveries multiplied and expanded knowledge, and suddenly doctors had the ability to cure the conditions that had been leading killers: infections and many communicable diseases. Antibiotics and vaccines revolutionized healthcare, vastly extended life expectancy, and redefined the role of medicine in everyday life.

## *When Did the Doctors Get Involved?*

Menopause entered the realm of medical care in the early 1940s, when researchers perfected the first estrogen pill. Called *Premarin,* the name under which the drug is still marketed today, this form of estrogen was manufactured from the urine of pregnant horses. Within a decade, millions of American women were taking this new miracle drug that made hot flashes, mood swings, and other undesirable signs of menopause go away. In fact, many women felt that with Premarin, they were going through "the change" with few noticeable changes at all.

In this new medical model of menopause, the normal indications of menopause suddenly became symptoms. Rather than asking ourselves whether

**Wise Up**

**Premarin** is the trade name for the estrogen-replacement drug marketed by Wyeth-Ayerst, a division of American Home Products Corporation. It is the second most commonly prescribed drug of any kind in the United States.

these were uncomfortable and disruptive or simply discomforting reminders that we're growing older, we focused attention and effort on eliminating them. Such actions are not without consequences, however—and sometimes the consequences are more serious than the circumstances we're trying to avoid.

## Can You Postpone the Body's Aging Process?

Premarin and the dozens of other hormone-replacement products (that we discuss in Part 4, "HRT or No HRT, That Is the Question") that have come on the market in the 50 years that doctors have been prescribing them for women going through menopause have helped revolutionize our thinking about fertility. If medical technology can so effectively minimize the manifestations of this significant life passage, can it delay or even prevent it? After all, new stories over the past few years have reported women in their 50s and even in their 60s who have given birth.

While postponing the body's aging processes to prolong fertility is an enticing possibility, we're not likely to see this as an alternative to aging for everyone. Women who conceive beyond what ordinarily would be menopause do so with the assistance of powerful fertility drugs (and often donor eggs), not estrogen replacement—this is a different matter altogether. Many questions remain about the long-term effects of using such drugs, as well as the long-term effects of estrogen replacements. No matter how closely these replacements mimic the natural estrogen that the human body produces, they're not quite the same. This is not to say that it might someday be possible to delay meno-pause indefinitely, but we need to learn more about what other effects this has and to better understand our reasons for doing it.

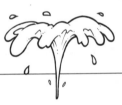

### Wellspring

The fact that researchers didn't discover a way to manufacture hormones until the early 1940s didn't keep doctors from attempting to alleviate the discomfort of their patients who were going through menopause. A book of medical advice published in the early 1900s offered a recipe combining ammonium bromide, potassium bromide, aromatic spirits of ammonia, and camphor water as a remedy for menopause. The woman was to take one spoonful three times a day by mouth until her symptoms subsided. There is no scientific reason this remedy would have any effect, although, of course, the signs of meno-pause would eventually abate, providing a sense of credibility.

## Menopause Is Not a Disease

Now women are looking at menopause with new eyes. Unlike our grandmothers and mothers, we know what medical technology can accomplish. We have options and decisions. Without discarding the advances that medical technology have made possible, we are reevaluating our passage through menopause. There is no question that modern medicine works wonders for the small percentage—about 20 percent—of women whose signs of menopause truly are symptoms that interfere with their lives. For everyone else, however, the true wonder might well be in enjoying the passage for what it is: a life transition. Despite nearly half a century of medical intervention, menopause is not a disease or even a health condition for most women. It is simply a stage in the normal life cycle of a woman.

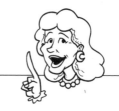

**Wise Woman's Wisdom**

"One is not born a woman, one becomes one."

—Simone de Beauvoir, *The Second Sex,* 1949

# Embracing Each Change of Life

Most of us have looked forward to certain transitions and changes in our lives. Physical milestones mark our progress through life. As infants, we smile, sit without support, and use our arms and legs to propel us, however inefficiently, from one location to another. We lose our baby teeth, grow and stretch, enter puberty, become young women with the potential to give birth, and start the cycle again for another human being. We and the people around us—family and friends—welcome and celebrate these transitions. Our passage through menopause should be a celebration of our path through life, past, present—and future!

---

### The Least You Need to Know

➤ Many myths and fallacies about menopause affect our perceptions of this life passage.

➤ Menopause is not a disease or a medical condition for most women, although some women may have problems during menopause that need medical attention.

➤ For more than 80 percent of women, the indications of menopause are mild and unobtrusive.

➤ Menopause is not the end of life for today's woman; it is the beginning of a new cycle in her life.

---

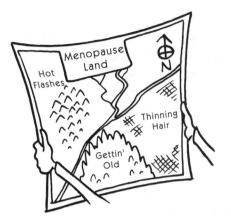

# Chapter 2

# Mapping Menopause: Facts, Folklore, and Fears

## In This Chapter

➤ The mythology of the crone goddess

➤ Menopause through history: facts and fables

➤ Menopause in the information age

➤ Living longer, living better

In many cultures, menstrual bleeding is both a physical and a symbolic discharge. In this view, as a woman passes the blood and tissues to complete her monthly menstrual cycle, she also passes knowledge and spirit. When menstruation ceases, in menopause, she retains knowledge and spirituality. This gives her a wisdom that grows with each month that she no longer menstruates. A woman well beyond menopause might be considered almost mystical.

Since it wasn't until the twentieth century that we had the technology to examine and understand the finer functions of the human body, mythology and folklore have become rooted in our experience. Although we now know the precise physiology of a woman's fertility cycle, myths and stories still add a dimension of timelessness to each woman's journey along that cycle.

# The Crone Goddess: Ancient Cultures Revere the Wise Woman

Mythology across cultures and times features the archetype of the triple goddess: the maiden, the mother, and the crone. The maiden represents the young virgin, ready to embark on the journey of her life. The mother represents reproduction and nurturing. The crone represents the culmination of life experience and wisdom.

In Greek mythology, the triple goddess archetype is the Fates, three women who sequentially control each person's life. Clotho, the maiden or the spinner, spins the thread that becomes the life. Lachesis, the mother or the "dispenser of lots," weaves the thread that Clotho spins into the life's destiny. Atropos, the crone, wields the shears that will cut the thread and end the life. Each Fate carries forward or grows from the actions of the other. Because the crone has the power to end life, she is the most revered and respected. It is her knowledge of the fabric that Lachesis weaves (as the life's destiny) that gives her insight into when to cut the thread. The other Fates are important, yes. But because Atropos holds the end of life in her hand, she also holds the continuation of life.

Ancient cultures greatly respected the wisdom and power of the crone, symbolically as well as in reality. In times when living beyond 40 or 50 years was in itself no small feat, those who continued even longer were viewed as having mystical gifts. It wasn't hard for an old woman to behave in ways that supported these beliefs: Because she had lived so many years, she did have much accumulated knowledge that made her appear wise and generous. Often, the wise crone would be the only one who knew how to remove a poisonous thorn or identify edible mushrooms.

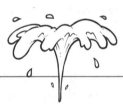

### Wellspring

Blood has long had mystical and symbolic meaning. In fact, it is the symbol of life itself, physically as well as spiritually, in nearly all cultures. Early Europeans believed that blood contained the essence of a person's soul. As a result, healing and magic practices often involved the ceremonial spilling (and sometimes drinking) of blood. This belief also gave rise to the legend of the devil demanding pacts be signed in blood so that he could return to claim the soul.

# Wisdom of the Ages: A History of Menopause

Many factors have affected menopause and our present knowledge of the experiences of women throughout history. In ancient times, when body functions were viewed as normal dimensions of nature, menstruation and menopause were simply elements of the cycle of life. There was nothing inherently good or bad about either. Over time, however, many cultures lost touch with the natural elements and cycles of life. Events that people didn't understand became attached to superstition and folklore. Misperceptions lead to fears. It has been a long journey through sometimes very dark times for womankind to reclaim the essence of what defines it.

## *Medieval Myths and Mysticism*

The 10 centuries or so that we now know as the Middle Ages (roughly 400 to 1500 B.C.E.) were times of struggle and need for everyone. Most people worked very hard just to survive. Food was often scarce, and disease was rampant. Warring tribes fought continually with each other in attempts to acquire more land, more property, and more resources. So few children lived to their first birthdays that most remained unnamed until they passed that milestone. Girls typically married as young as age 10 and nearly always by age 13 or 14. Given the difficult and numerous challenges of the times, many women were widowed by age 20, grandmothers by age 30, and buried by age 50.

Medieval perceptions of menstruation and menopause were largely mystical. Common belief equated menstruation in the woman to ejaculation in the man, a physiological release of sexual tension. Menstrual blood was also an essential component of conception, combining with the man's sperm to produce new life. When a woman's periods stopped during pregnancy, according to the sages of the time, it was so that the "menstruum" (considered the woman's seed) could feed and sustain the growing fetus. Of course, the writings of the time advised that this accumulation also fed the woman's sexual desire, generating the need for frequent sexual activity (as long as it wasn't an eclipse of the moon, that is—legend had it that having sexual intercourse with a menstruating woman during a lunar eclipse would most certainly bring disease or death).

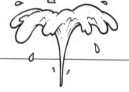

**Wellspring**

Word origins are not always precise. Most dictionaries cite the probable root word of *crone* as the French *carogne*, which means "carrion" (dead or rotting flesh). Yet they speculate that *crony*, which means "old friend," is derived from the Greek word *chronios*, meaning "long lasting."

Not surprisingly in a time when there was little knowledge or understanding of the human body, menstrual blood was considered poisonous despite its assumed role in procreation. According to the scientists of the time, contact with it could dull the edge of a steel blade, shrivel the fruit on trees, sour wine, and make dogs go mad. So strong was the power of a menstruating woman, in fact, that a single look from her could kill all the bees in a hive! Menstruating women were not permitted to work in the fields, butcher meat, churn butter, or engage in nearly any of the routine tasks that ordinarily occupied their lives.

It appears that few women really enjoyed any respite, however—most were pregnant nearly continuously during their childbearing years. Unfortunately, there was little for those who survived years of pregnancy and childbirth to look forward to at menopause. Rather than being welcomed or even understood as a normal life transition, menopause was a suspicious event that occurred without apparent cause. The revered crone of ancient times was looked upon in medieval times as a witch and often was persecuted or killed. Little wonder that this era was once known as the Dark Ages!

## Mona Lisa: Life in the High Renaissance

Many ponder the whimsical smile of one of history's most famous women, captured for eternity in the brilliant brush strokes of Leonardo da Vinci, a free-thinking artist who broke with convention not just in painting, but in science and medicine as well. The painting is actually a portrait of the wife of another Renaissance artist, Francesco del Giocondo, and is also known as "la Gioconda." Aside from tantalizing viewers for centuries, the Mona Lisa changed the way artists painted and people viewed women.

What most people know about the Renaissance is that it's hard to spell. But this period in time, from the French word for *rebirth,* was one of the most dynamic and exciting eras in modern history. Emerging from the darkness of the Middle Ages in the fourteenth century, there was a sense of exuberance and awakening. Dance, music, art, science, and intellectual pursuits—luxuries for so many centuries—again flourished. Although the Renaissance was a relatively short era compared to the 1,000 years of the Middle Ages, this 200-year period brought about great change in living conditions as well as in perceptions and understanding.

New knowledge of the human body and its functions gave rise to new and more positive understanding of the menstrual cycle. In 1561, Italian anatomist Gabriele Fallopius (1523–1562) discovered the tubes branching from the top of the uterus and arching downward toward the ovaries, which we now call the fallopian tubes. A little more than 100 years later, in 1668, Dutch scientist Regnier de Graaf (1641–1673) completed the basic understanding of how conception occurs when he identified and described the ovary and the egg-containing follicles covering its surface (although it would be another 90 years before the microscope made it possible to actually identify ova, or eggs).

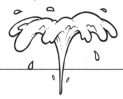

### Wellspring

Until relatively modern times, childbirth was a leading cause of death among women. Unsanitary living conditions, poor nutrition, and misunderstanding about the female body and the process of birth all contributed to the risks. Although records are not consistent, it appears that about one-fourth to one-half of women who died young died in childbirth or from its complications. Bleeding and infection were the primary problems. Not until the discovery of sulfa and penicillin in the 1940 did pregnancy cease to be a potentially life-threatening experience.

## The Victorian Era: Button Up

By all accounts, Queen Victoria was a powerful and dominating ruler. All good things must come to an end, though, and this monarch of England seemed to make it her personal mission to see that at least those of the Renaissance era did. After ascending to the throne in 1837, Queen Victoria established rules for every aspect of living. Temperance, piety, and high moral tone replaced the exuberance and exploration of the two preceding centuries. Public behavior was polite to the point of excluding recognition of any and all unpleasantries. Private behavior was just that: No one talked about anything that wasn't acceptable public behavior. And publicly, body functions didn't exist.

The prim and proper façade that characterized the Victorian time was a great disservice to women. In keeping with the sense of modesty at the time, women did not appear unclothed in front of male doctors. Yet male doctors were rapidly taking over the practice of delivering babies, previously the province of female midwives. Despite the amazing discoveries of the Renaissance, there was still significant misunderstanding about the female body and its functioning, especially during pregnancy and childbirth. And since no one talked—at least not openly—about problems and difficulties, women felt tremendously isolated.

## What's It All Got to Do with *You?*

So here we are, stepping into the twenty-first century. How does the past have anything to do with the future? Again we come back to cycles. We are in a contemporary renaissance of sorts, a time when there is great openness about sexuality and

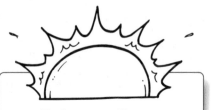

## Embracing Change

In cities across America, women's groups are again embracing the power of storytelling through sharing their menopause and aging experiences. Many also incorporate elements of ritual—symbolically welcoming wrinkles, for example—to celebrate the changes that menopause brings into their lives.

reproduction. Women talk often with each other, and with men, about PMS, pregnancy, mood swings, hot flashes, and other formerly taboo topics. We are seeing a return to the wise woman perspective, with honor and respect for women in general and older women in particular. As more women pass through menopause, there is a greater interest in understanding the transition from medical, social, and spiritual contexts.

We are coming full circle, returning to a sense of wonder and awe about the cycle of the feminine. During the glory years of medical intervention (roughly the 1960s through the 1990s), we viewed menopause as a problem or condition requiring treatment. At the same time, we dismissed and even scorned the folklore and stories that previous generations of women relied on to guide them through the passage of menopause. Now we recognize that much of what such passages embody is symbolic or representational. Of course, there are physical elements of menopause—it is a physical event, as much as anything. But rather than being misrepresentations, stories and folklore can share a common experience across generations and across cultures.

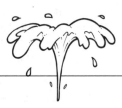

## Wellspring

Although ultimately the term "Victorian" came to be synonymous with repression and restriction in both actions and attitudes, Queen Victoria (1819–1901) herself could well be considered a pioneer in women's equality. She came to power at a time when women rulers were rare, and two years later she proposed to the cousin who would become her husband, Prince Albert. During their marriage, Queen Victoria turned over the keys to the government, so to speak, to Prince Albert and focused her attention on raising their nine children. But Prince Albert died unexpectedly young, leaving Queen Victoria a widow at age 42. Thrust back into the spotlight of leadership, Queen Victoria became a knowledgeable yet controlling leader.

# Fast-Forward to the Information Age

Our mothers learned what they knew about menopause from their mothers and aunts, who learned what they knew from their mothers and aunts. So it has been through much of history: One generation educates and enlightens the next. Until now. Today's women have more information literally at their fingertips than anyone even dreamed would be possible 20 years ago. But now, anyone who has access to a personal computer and the Internet can learn about the latest research findings even before the studies hit publication.

The information age we live in is a mixed blessing. On the one hand, it's great to get the newest knowledge with a few mouse clicks. On the other hand, it's often difficult to sort out which information is accurate and which is unsubstantiated or even quackery. Researchers sometimes rush to publication knowing that if they don't announce their findings, someone else will. The result is a confusing array of reports and recommendations that often conflict with one another. How's a woman to know what information to trust?

The answer, unfortunately, is that sometimes she can't. It's important to seek reputable resources, such as respected professional journals that require published studies to be *peer-reviewed*. Although this is not a guarantee that a study's findings are reliable and sound, it's a strong indication that the researchers followed accepted practices in designing and carrying out the study. The public library is a good resource for locating medical journals that publish peer-reviewed articles, as are Web sites such as www.medscape.com. If you have questions about information you come across, ask your doctor.

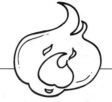

**Hot Flash!**

Know your sources when you do your research on the Internet! Most people don't intentionally post incorrect information on their Web sites. However, many people do post accounts of their personal experiences and opinions. It can be difficult to distinguish between these sites and those that provide generally accepted advice and information.

**Wise Up**

**Peer review** is a formal process through which professionals of comparable expertise assess a study's methods and structures for reliability and scientific soundness.

Technology is growing like dandelions in June. So, too, is the new information it spawns. Techniques and methods not available just a few years ago can yield results that turn conventional wisdom upside down. New knowledge upends what has become common practice. In 1990, for example, doctors and women alike believed that menopause was a 10- to 15-year transition best "treated" to minimize or suppress its signs and symptoms. We now know that menopause itself lasts just two to three years and that many women experience a transition into menopause called perimenopause. And we're rethinking what needs treatment and intervention, and what needs recognition, understanding, and acceptance.

## Can You Ever Be Too Rich, Too Thin ... or Too Young?

Ah, too much. Does it exist? Many of us would shout "no!" in a heartbeat—at least when the question pertains to what we perceive as positives. Who wouldn't want to have more money than they could possibly spend or to never have to worry about getting on a scale? But technology and its potential raise interesting dilemmas for today's women. Just because we can delay—and may someday be able to prevent—menopause, should we? If at age 45 the average woman can expect to live another 30 to 40 years, is there any reason *not* to use the tools available to modern medicine to intercede in Mother Nature's cycle?

It seems that as life expectancy extends, the cycles of life should broaden correspondingly. With a projected life span of 90 years or longer, it makes sense that menstruation and menopause would start later in life. This could shift the cycle of fertility ahead by as much as a decade, letting women start their families when they're more mature and they've established their career paths. Wouldn't that be great?

Mother Nature doesn't seem to think so, and in fact is making at least one shift in the opposite direction. Across cultures, girls today start menstruating about five years earlier than did their counterparts a century ago. But women enter menopause at the same age they have for nearly all of recorded history. A woman's fertile years are extending, yes, although not necessarily to match her lengthening life span.

Despite our ability to alter some of the human body's physical functions, researchers have yet to discover any magic elixir or technological miracle that can keep us forever young. This raises philosophical, ethical, social, and practical concerns about approaches that delay specific physiological inevitabilities. And for many of these concerns, there are no easy answers. No one really knows where today's decisions will lead.

# 100 Years Ago, Women Didn't Live to Be 100!

Certainly women have been living beyond menopause for quite some time. But at no time in history have so many of them done so for so many years. One hundred years ago, the average American woman could expect to reach the ripe old age of 55, barely long enough to complete her passage through menopause. Today's woman entering menopause around age 50 can anticipate another three or four decades of healthful living, and a girl born in the year 2000 can expect to live well into her 90s. Indeed, there are already more nonagenarians (people in their 90s) living today than ever in recorded history, and their age group is growing faster than any other.

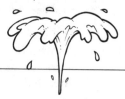

### Wellspring

Throughout much of recorded history, it has been the role of the grandmother to assist with childrearing responsibilities and to step in and take over if the mother became seriously ill or died. In cultures that predate structured society—the era of hunters and gatherers—there is evidence that grandmothers played a far more involved role in raising children than did fathers. Some modern cultures have formalized this role by having a widowed grandmother move in with the family to help with the kids in exchange for the family taking care of her needs.

## Baby Boomers Break the Age Barrier

You can blame it all on the Baby Boomers. This population group, born between 1946 and 1964, is the single largest such group in American history. More than 75 million babies were born in this post-war boom, and they are entering midlife and menopause in numbers large enough to change the demographic structure of the country—as well as our attitudes about aging. This has focused significant attention on matters related to growing older, from gray hair to hot flashes.

If you're in this age group, you no doubt already have a sense of this from the advertisements you see on television and receive through the mail. Baby Boomers are suddenly a marketing gold mine as retailers realize that they are rapidly representing the largest share of consumer sales. This is actually good news. For the first time in this country's history (and for a long time in general), it's not only fashionable, but also desirable to be older! As the numbers of people over age 50 continue to grow, everyone from savvy merchandisers to astute politicians are taking notice and catering to their needs and interests. Your journey through menopause need not be the isolated experience of your mother's or grandmother's generation. You have more company and more information than ever before.

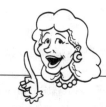

### Wise Woman's Wisdom

"By the age of 50 you have made yourself what you are, and if it is good, it is better than your youth."

—Marya Mannes, *More in Anger*, 1958

## You May Spend as Much Time Over 40 as Under

The generations of women before us tended to look at menopause as the gateway to The End. After menopause, it was all downhill. And admittedly, if the odds were that you'd only live another 8 to 10 years, there was a fair amount of truth to this perception. That no doubt shaped how women felt about "the change"—if you knew it was your last passage, wouldn't you go through it kicking and screaming, fingernails ripping through the walls of time as you struggled to evade the inevitable?

If you're near enough to menopause that you're reading everything about it that you can get your hands on, relax. Take a slow, deep breath. You're not dying! You're entering the last half of your life, to be sure. But *half* is the operative word here. Women who are right now 40 to 45 years old are truly in the middle of their lives. And the 40 to 45 years that you have left is a long time to waste kicking, screaming, and resisting! In fact, it's a long time to enjoy the parts of life that you haven't had time to enjoy until now. A midlife crisis happens for a reason—to open your eyes to the joys that still lie ahead of you.

## Coming of Age, Coming into Our Own

Most women identify the years after menopause as the most enjoyable time of their lives. They feel comfortable and confident about themselves. They know that life is too short to sweat the small stuff—and for many, this knowledge becomes freedom.

---

### The Least You Need to Know

➤ In many cultures throughout history, menopause has been a time of reverence and status.

➤ Misunderstanding about menstruation and menopause has led to much misinformation that has given these elements of a woman's life cycle an undeserved negative image.

➤ Although we now know far more about the functions of the human body than did previous generations, a lot of misinformation and misunderstanding still circulate.

➤ While women have always lived long enough to experience menopause, never before have they lived so long *beyond* menopause.

---

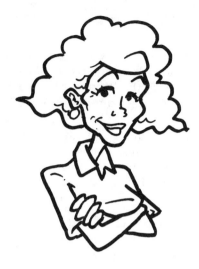

# Chapter 3

# The Power of the Second Spring

---

## In This Chapter

➤ Examining how we age

➤ How supplements affect (and don't affect) the aging process

➤ How you feel about menopause: a self-exploration

➤ The many faces of beauty

➤ How to feel young even as you're growing older

---

It has often been said that beginnings and endings are one and the same. As one experience or event ends, another begins—even if it's not obvious to you at the time. Such is the cycle of life. The conclusion of one stage is the start of the next. Menarche (the start of menstruation) marks the end of childhood and the beginning of motherhood and fertility (actual or symbolic) in a woman's life, or the transition from maiden to mother. Menopause marks the end of caring for others and the beginning of caring for the self, or the transition from mother to crone or wise woman.

Menopause also marks the beginning of a new era in life, a time in which many women discover (or rediscover) creativity and freedom. This "second spring" is often a time of new and unexpected growth. You might start a new business, take up painting or writing, travel to exotic locations, or decide to become a foster parent. With many of the challenges of "making it" finally out of the way, there is time and energy to finally focus on what matters to you. Many women enter this second spring with a renewed sense of who they are and what they aim to accomplish with their lives.

# Age Will Not Be Defied

For as long as people have realized the connection between aging and mortality, they have searched for ways to delay both. The Spanish explorer Ponce de Leon (1460–1521) discovered the state of Florida on a quest in search of the legendary Fountain of Youth believed to be on Bimini Island in the Bahamas. Other cultures have tried potions, rituals, and other practices in the effort to remain forever young. All such efforts have been to no avail, although this doesn't keep us from trying. Even today, advertisements touting health and beauty products that promise to give at least the impression of more youthful looks crowd the pages of magazines. Turn back the clock, erase wrinkles, get younger, healthier-looking skin—the appeal is hard to resist in a culture that worships youth.

Regardless of our efforts to push it back, however, aging marches onward in our lives. Some people naturally show little sign of increasing age—their hair remains dark and full, their faces stay smooth and clear, their backs stand tall and straight. No one really knows what determines how we age. What we do know is that everyone does age. Aging is living.

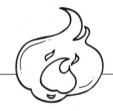

### Hot Flash!

The U.S. Food and Drug Administration (FDA) banned DHEA in 1985, prohibiting it from being sold in the United States. However, the substance re-emerged as a dietary supplement after the 1994 Federal Dietary Supplement Health and Education Act exempted such products from the FDA's effectiveness and safety testing requirements.

## Supplements to Reverse Aging: Do They Work?

Numerous products marketed as dietary or nutritional supplements claim to stop or reverse the aging process. One over-the-counter product, known as DHEA (dehydroepiandrosterone), has long been touted as a miracle substance that can do everything from build muscle mass to boost immunity, burn fat, and improve memory. None of these claims has been substantiated in scientific studies, but such studies have demonstrated the potential for serious side effects, including liver damage and an increased risk of heart disease and certain cancers. DHEA does occur naturally in the human body in youth, with production peaking around age 25. After this time, natural DHEA levels drop to nearly nil fairly quickly. This has led to conclusions that there is a correlation between DHEA and other changes that take place in the body as it ages. When taken as a supplement, DHEA is converted by the body into estrogen and testosterone.

Another hormone product available without a prescription is melatonin. Melatonin also occurs naturally in the body (produced by the brain) and appears to have the primary function of regulating sleep cycles. Some people use melatonin supplements to ease insomnia, though it appears to be more effective when used to cope with jet lag or sleep/wake rhythm problems. Doctors are still exploring the relationship of melatonin to the human daily circadian rhythm. Ask your doctor before taking melatonin. No studies have yet demonstrated that melatonin can affect the aging process, enhance sex drive, or fight cancer, other claims now surfacing for this supplement.

Many people take vitamin and mineral supplements, especially those called *antioxidants,* to bolster immunity, slow aging, and protect against certain diseases such as heart disease, cancer, and *Alzheimer's disease*. Vitamin E is the most popular of these, and likely the most effective. Several studies question the effectiveness of another common antioxidant, beta carotene (which your body converts to vitamin A). More research also is needed to determine whether substances such as vitamin C, selenium (a mineral common in seafood), and coenzyme $Q_{10}$ (an antioxidant naturally produced

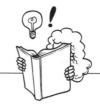

**Wise Up**

An **antioxidant** is a substance that neutralizes free radicals, the natural byproducts of metabolism. **Alzheimer's disease** is a progressive, incurable condition in which the nerve cells in the brain degenerate, resulting in loss of cognitive (thinking) ability and memory.

by the human body) are as effective in supplement form as they appear to be when ingested by eating the fruits and vegetables that contain them. Yet while vitamin and mineral supplements aren't likely to do you any harm when taken as instructed, they probably don't do all that their labels and advertising claim. Some nutritional supplements are both important and helpful, of course. Although we think we eat well, our diets often fall short when it comes to key nutrients such as calcium and the B vitamins.

## To Long for Youth Is to Forego the Future

"It's a poor sort of memory that only works backwards," comments the Queen to Alice in Lewis Carroll's classic *Alice's Adventures in Wonderland*. Yet it does. Memory is like a rear-view mirror, displaying the scenery of our lives in retrospect. And this is good. After all, the past builds the future. Where looking backward becomes more of a problem than a pleasant reverie is when we long to live in the view we see. Like the triple goddess—maiden, mother, and crone—we are the accumulation of our experiences. Each stage in life comes from the one before. Even if you could go back to an earlier time in your life, the experience wouldn't be what you remember. Memory tends to be selective: We recall extremes of joy and sorrow, and we often blur the events in between.

Do you remember when all you wanted to be was older? You wanted to be old enough to drive, to date, to work, to drink, to vote, to marry, to have children of your own. You looked to the future with eagerness and anticipation because the future held all the good things in life. Now that you're living the future you dreamed about when you were younger, of course, the view's a little different. Days, weeks, and months that dragged into years when you were young and waiting for them to arrive now flash past as years. But just as you might wish that you had spent more time enjoying the present when you were younger, you may someday find yourself feeling the same way about *this* present when it becomes your past. So if you want to go back, go back to looking ahead!

## A Gateway to New Life Experience

Many of our perceptions about menopause come from people we've known during their passages through this life transition—grandmothers, mothers, aunts, sisters, friends, neighbors, or even co-workers. While there are certain universal elements to the transition—every woman's period stops, for example—there are also many differences.

Think of it as being similar to taking a trip by car to a destination you've heard about but never visited, yet all your friends have been there. Each friend will tell you something different about both the trip and the destination. One might recall the scenery seen through the car window, while another might remember only that there were no bathrooms for 200 miles. One might describe the destination as exciting and busy, while another might grumble that it was loud and distracting. Each person traveled the same route in a similar vehicle and arrived at the same location, yet they all had entirely different experiences.

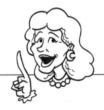

### Wise Woman's Wisdom

"What becomes of lost opportunities? Perhaps our guardian angel gathers them up and will give them back when we've grown wiser—and will use them rightly."

—Helen Keller

So it is with menopause—and all life transitions, really. What your experience is depends to a great extent on how you shape it. Of course, you cannot control your journey's bumps, jolts, and detours. You might flush with hot flashes or snap at someone when you didn't realize that you were feeling so irritable, just as your car could have a flat tire on a road trip even though you carefully checked each tire's tread and air pressure before leaving.

What you can control, however, is how you respond to such events. When a tire goes flat, you pull over, rummage through the trunk to locate all the jack pieces the manufacturer has tucked away in odd little spaces, and change the tire. You can swear and stomp and slam. You can sing and dance and laugh. Either way, the spare replaces the flat. All you can direct is how you respond. In either case, the event becomes part of your journey. So it is with menopause.

# How Do *You* Feel About Menopause? A Self-Exploration

How you feel about menopause has a significant effect on how you will experience it. What (and who) has shaped your perspectives and views? This self-exploration can help you discover what your feelings really are. There are no right or wrong answers, so just jot down your responses on the lines (or on a separate sheet of paper, if you don't want to write in your book).

1. My first exposure to menopause was when ...

   _____

   _____

2. The first words I remember hearing anyone use to describe menopause were ...

   _____

   _____

3. The one thing I remember most clearly about my mother's menopause experience (or that of other significant adult woman) is ...

   _____

   _____

4. When I think of myself going through menopause, the first words that come to mind are ...

   _____

   _____

5. When I think of myself growing older, the first images that come to mind are ...

   _____

   _____

6. I believe that menopause will change my life for the better in these three ways ...

   _____

   _____

7. I believe that menopause will change my life for the worse in these three ways ...

   _____

   _____

8. My greatest fear about menopause is ...

   _____

   _____

9. What I most eagerly anticipate about menopause is ...

_____

_____

10. The problems I expect to have during menopause include ...

_____

_____

11. The people I know I can count on to understand and support me on my journey through menopause include ...

_____

_____

12. My partner's feelings about menopause are ...

_____

_____

13. What I think will change the most in my life following menopause is ...

_____

_____

14. What I think will change the least in my life following menopause is ...

_____

_____

15. I expect my menopause experience to be ...

_____

_____

# Changing the Face of Beauty

What do you see when you look in the mirror? Does the image that stares back at you startle you or please you? One of the paradoxes of growing older is that we don't feel any different than we did at, say, age 30. But our bodies and our appearances *are* changing, even if we still feel the same.

Ideals, standards, and tastes change not only with the whims of fad and fashion, but also on a personal level as our lives change and evolve. Chances are, what appealed to you when you were 25 is not what you'll admire when you're 45, 65, or 85, whether that's clothing and cars, or careers and people. Just for fun, make a quick list of the 10 most important things in your life when you were 25, as you best remember them, and now. How many are the same?

## Draw a Picture of a Beautiful Woman

Nothing is more subjective than our perceptions of beauty. To some, youthful innocence is the embodiment of beauty. Others see beauty in the lines and wrinkles of a wise and experienced face. What you define as beautiful has as much to do with what you like as what you don't like, and what emotions the two evoke. What do you see in your mind's eye when you envision the ideal woman? How does she compare to the woman you see in the mirror—not the face that greets you when you first wake up, but the one that peers back at you when you're doing that last check before leaving the house? Are you surprised, perhaps, to discover that she's really not so different from the ideal in your mind?

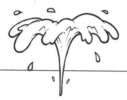

### Wellspring

The supermodel ideal so prevalent today is a manifestation of modern tastes. Until Twiggy burst onto the modeling scene in the early 1960s, models were a relatively fair representation of the average American woman. They wore close to the same dress size and had similar proportions. Since Twiggy, the gap between the supermodel ideal and real life has steadily increased. While a supermodel struts the latest fashions in a size 2, the typical American woman struggles to fit into a size 14.

## Who, You, Old? No ...

As the saying goes, you're only as old as you feel. Although some mornings you may crawl out of bed feeling older than Methuselah, more often than not you probably feel pretty much the same as you did when you were in your 30s. Rejoice! There's nothing wrong with feeling younger than you are. In fact, it goes a long way toward creating and maintaining a positive sense of self and a healthful outlook on life. If you feel young, you likely have numerous and diverse activities going on in your life. You spend time with other people as well as with yourself, enjoy your work (whether in an office or in a garden), and have hobbies or interests that you indulge in simply because you enjoy them.

Odds are, you're also fairly active. You at least walk regularly, and you probably have an exercise routine that provides aerobic exercise three times a week or so. Perhaps you jog, do dance aerobics, ride a bicycle, walk, or run on a treadmill. If this describes your life, you may have discovered the closest thing to a fountain of youth: exercise.

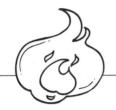

### Hot Flash!

Products and treatments that promise to turn back the clock are not without risk. Medications, chemical peels, collagen injections, and surgery are both costly and ultimately temporary. Be sure that you have a realistic sense of the potential benefits before you move forward with such alterations.

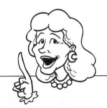

### Wise Woman's Wisdom

"When she stopped conforming to the conventional picture of femininity, she finally began to enjoy being a woman."

—Betty Friedan, *The Feminine Mystique,* 1963

Regular exercise strengthens muscle and bone, improves balance, and maintains weight. It also makes you feel better, both in general and about yourself. You think more clearly, are less tired, and remember more. Even if younger is not what you're after, exercise does your body and your mind good.

# Being Proactive About Menopause

Although it's true that you can't control your menopause experience, you can most certainly shape it, starting with your attitude and your beliefs. Consider menopause as you would consider any grand adventure or life change. Preparation is empowerment. The best way to confront your fears is to learn as much as you can. Make a plan for using your knowledge. Think about what is important to you and how you might handle potential problems and challenges. Find out how your primary healthcare provider feels about menopause. Do you have health problems that could complicate your passage? Make an appointment to discuss your worries and concerns.

If you've needed to make some changes in your life but have been resisting them, consider menopause as a catalyst. After all, menopause is a time of transition. It is a natural opportunity to make changes to improve your life. Don't change just for the sake of change, of course. But think about where you are in your life. Are you in a job that you don't enjoy? Start looking at options. Do you eat nutritiously and exercise regularly? If not, this is as good a time as any to start doing both. All that you do to ease your journey through menopause can become the patterns you follow for the rest of your life, if you let them.

## *Staring Down Media Stereotypes*

The supermodel look so popular today is a stark contrast to the reality of most women. Their lithe and lean bodies appear almost androgynous, with slender limbs, narrow hips, and small breasts. They weigh barely 75 percent of what the average American woman weighs. While fewer than 5 percent of American women have a similar body type, nearly 95 percent of them want the look anyway. Most health experts agree that it's an unhealthful desire.

There are two reasons for this. The first is that superthin supermodels often weigh significantly less than health standards say they should. Rather than representing the ideal body weight and proportions, the typical supermodel presents the image of an undernourished body. The second is that it's hard to appreciate yourself for who and what you are when you're trying so hard to be something else. You are far better off if you can appreciate your body for what it is. Eat nutritiously, exercise regularly, and forget about looking like that model on the magazine cover!

And as more women decide to accept themselves for the size 12, or 14 (the American average), or 16, or more that they are, retailers and advertisers are wising up. Many stores feature a broader range of sizes, including "plus" sizes, and use models with more realistic and representative proportions. This acceptance seems easier as we grow older and our bodies drift farther from the media ideal. Perhaps we just become more accepting and less pressured to be what we're not and what we really don't want to be. Although aging can produce physical changes that we don't like, such as arthritis, most people feel more comfortable with their bodies and themselves by the time they hit midlife.

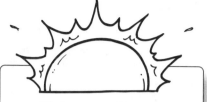

**Embracing Change**

Contrary to advertising hype, men tend to be more attracted to women who display strong signs of fertility: broader hips and fuller breasts. Attraction also changes with maturity, as the package becomes far less important than its contents. Men and women both tend to seek partners with whom they feel strong emotional and spiritual connections.

## Putting Your Best Face Forward

No matter how you look, what's important is that you feel good about it. Sometimes you need an attitude readjustment, a recognition that you are who you are and that's who you should be. Accepting yourself gives you a sense of inner peace and confidence that shows. When you like your appearance, not because it aligns with some external and arbitrary standard but because you feel good about how you look, then you look good.

## The Least You Need to Know

➤ Aging is inevitable, and we can't change that. What we can change is how we feel about it.

➤ Supplements and products that promise to halt or reverse aging typically lack the evidence to support their claims.

➤ Although every woman experiences menopause, every woman's experience of menopause is unique.

➤ Our ideals, standards, and tastes change as we grow older.

➤ The closest thing to a fountain of youth is regular exercise.

# Part 2
# Midlife Metamorphosis

*You know, from countless vacations and business trips, that getting ready for the journey that lies ahead is often more intense than the journey itself. Although there are no suitcases to pack or plugged-in coffee makers to worry about, menopause is no different—except that, when you return, it's not to the same old life you left behind. Yes, many familiar trappings remain. But you won't be the person you were before embarking on this midlife adventure. These preparations are for a trip that will take you to a new and exciting point in your life.*

*The next five chapters discuss issues that you might find yourself confronting as your body readies itself for the journey of a lifetime.*

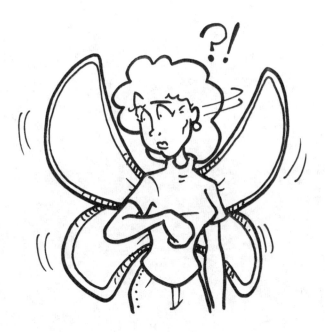

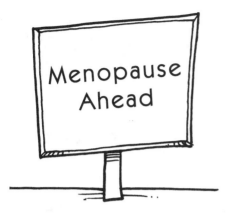

# Chapter 4

# Perimenopause: Approaching Menopause

---

### In This Chapter

➤ Understanding the distinction between perimenopause and menopause

➤ The relationship between PMS and perimenopause

➤ What's happening with your hormones

➤ Using birth control pills during perimenopause

➤ How to take care of yourself in this time of transition

---

Not so long ago, doctors and women alike believed that menopause was an event that could span a decade or longer. But recent research suggests that menopause is a singular event—a woman's last menstrual period—identified retrospectively. What we had come to accept as the menopause experience is really a two-stage process—the events and changes leading to menopause, and menopause itself.

Most of what we perceive as the discomforts of menopause are actually events related to physical preparations for the end of fertility. Just as it took several years for our bodies to gear up for fertility, it takes several years for the functions of fertility to wind down.

## The Progress of Understanding

Before doctors discovered the relationship between hormones, ovulation, and menstruation, they believed that a woman's body just suddenly ceased to be fertile. The irregular periods that are a hallmark of menopause signaled the onset of this ending.

Doctors believed that menopause was a fairly brief and distinctive event, although not quite as prompt as turning off a switch. From about the 1950s until the 1990s, the common understanding of menopause shifted to the belief that a woman's body gradually decreased hormone production beginning around age 35. By age 50, the decline was pronounced enough that hormone levels were no longer high enough to initiate ovulation, bringing menstrual cycles to a stop. Rather than being the fairly straight on/off switch that doctors perceived in earlier centuries, menopause was instead seen more like a dimmer switch, gradually shutting down the flow of hormones.

By the early 1990s, scientists had developed highly sophisticated and sensitive tests that could precisely measure hormone levels and activity. From these measures, doctors learned that their common understanding wasn't quite correct. There were two distinct and different stages to what had previously been viewed as the single event of menopause.

During the first of these stages, perimenopause, hormone levels do begin changing when a woman is in her late 30s or early 40s. But they don't do so with any pattern or consistency, or gradually as though being shut down with a dimmer switch. Instead, they fluctuate wildly, as though under the control of a mischievous child randomly flashing the switch on and off.

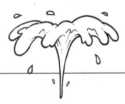

### Wellspring

In 1902, the physiologist Ernest Starling (1866–1927) isolated the first hormone identified in the human body, the intestinal hormone secretin. The discovery gave new insight into the often mysterious workings of the human body. By the second half of the twentieth century, scientists had discovered more than 50 different hormones, including those that regulate sexuality and reproduction. Our knowledge of how hormones work remains incomplete, although it's clear that they are part of an intricate and delicate biochemical balance that affects nearly every function in the body.

# When It's More Than Really Bad PMS

Is it *PMS*, or is it menopause? If you're in your 40s, it could be neither—or both. Doctors now recognize that there is a distinct period of time in the years preceding menopause during which a woman's body is beginning preparations to transition into menopause. This time is called *perimenopause* and can extend from 3 to 15 years, although the average is 3 to 6 years. During perimenopause, you still have periods, although they might become less regular. Pregnancy is less common but still possible. You also may experience mood swings, hot flashes, and other signs of menopause. You haven't yet entered menopause, although your life path is taking you closer.

**Wise Up**

**PMS,** or premenstrual syndrome, is a collection of symptoms that begin after ovulation and that usually conclude when menstruation begins. **Perimenopause** is the time of transition between a woman's childbearing years and the cessation of menstruation.

## Signs and Symptoms of Perimenopause

The signs and symptoms of perimenopause often resemble a cross between PMS and menopause. A woman in her late 30s or early 40s might ovulate one month and produce a viable egg, and then not ovulate for several months yet still have apparently normal periods. Or, she might experience several months of unusually painful and heavy periods, followed by several months of irregular and light periods. She could have wide and dramatic mood swings, night sweats, and hot flashes. She might have trouble sleeping, tire more easily, and lose interest in sex. She could also experience symptoms more like those of PMS, such as fluid retention, headache, backache, and lower abdominal cramps or pain.

## The Relationship Between PMS and Perimenopause

Some women experience a worsening of PMS, or experience PMS for the first time, as they enter perimenopause—almost a "worst of both worlds" circumstance. Not only are they continuing to menstruate, but their bodies are also preparing for menopause. The resulting hormonal turmoil appears to upset the body's biochemical balance. Most doctors believe that this imbalance generates the range and intensity of often unpleasant physical and emotional symptoms that some women experience.

## Charting Your Period Patterns

One way to gauge what is happening with your body is to begin charting your periods and any symptoms that you have. This doesn't have to be an elaborate project, just a brief written record to reveal any sort of pattern. You can jot notes on a calendar or create a journal where you can write more extensively about your thoughts, emotions, and physical experiences. This will help both you and your healthcare provider determine whether you are entering perimenopause or dealing with PMS— or both—and then choose an appropriate course of action.

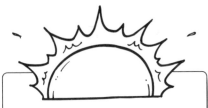

# Oh, Those Fluctuating Hormones!

If you sometimes feel like your body is at war with itself, you're not far off the mark. For most of your adult life, up until now, your body has enjoyed a fairly stable balance of hormones that kept it functioning in a regular and predictable fashion. Think of it like a finely geared clock. As long as all the gears move and rotate at the speeds and in the directions of their design, the clock's movement is smooth and quiet, and its time is accurate. But what happens if one gear suddenly reverses direction or speeds to four times its usual rate? All the other gears, being interlocked with the errant wheel, also reverse or speed up. Because their movements are synchronized, however, the efforts to adjust simply result in chaos.

What happens within your body during perimenopause is very similar. All the hormones are flowing along just as they should, and then suddenly one spikes. This triggers responses in the others, like the clock gears. By the time the hormone levels have all shifted, however, the one that spiked has returned to normal. So now you have all these other hormones at irregular levels. Your confused body doesn't know how to react to the conflicting messages it's receiving, and the result is a bewildering set of actions that are themselves in conflict. What's a woman to do?

**Embracing Change**

If you are taking birth control pills or have polycystic ovary syndrome (PCOS), it will be difficult for you to tell when you are entering perimenopause. The hormones in birth control pills offset any natural fluctuations in your body. Irregular periods and altered hormone levels are key symptoms of PCOS, which can be present during a woman's entire reproductive years.

## Perimenopause Is Not Early Menopause

Because the signs of perimenopause often resemble those of menopause, many women assume that perimenopause is just an early stage of menopause. It is not. Most women continue menstruating during perimenopause, although their periods usually become irregular and often unpredictable. Their ovaries are still producing enough follicle-stimulating hormone (FSH) to initiate the release of an egg each month (or at least some months). And while the quality of eggs during perimenopause is poor (meaning that they are beginning to deteriorate), they are often still viable (capable of fertilization).

Although we view the cessation of menstruation as the marker of menopause, from a clinical perspective menopause occurs when the ovaries stop functioning (which shows itself by ending menstruation). In perimenopause, the ovaries are still functioning. In early menopause, the ovaries have stopped functioning at an earlier age than is typical. Doctors can usually, although not always, tell from FSH and other hormone levels whether this is what's happening.

## Dealing with the Storm in Your Body

There are many approaches to coping with and managing the hormonal turmoil that's stirring up a storm in your body. Some women find it enough to know that what they're experiencing is a normal, albeit frustrating, dimension of the transition they are entering. They decide to just live with their symptoms, knowing that the problems are transient and will disappear as menopause continues. Other women find their lives sufficiently disrupted that they prefer some sort of intervention. The only choice that's right is the one that works for you.

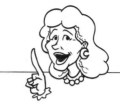

**Wise Woman's Wisdom**

"I'm not having hot flashes. I'm having power surges."

—Bumper sticker

# Should You Take Hormones for Perimenopause?

The signs and symptoms of perimenopause are severe enough for some women that they interfere with daily life. When this is the case, hormone treatment is likely to provide relief. This commonly takes the form of either hormone replacement therapy (HRT) or birth control pills. As long as a woman is clearly perimenopausal and still ovulating, most doctors recommend birth control pills. A woman who is close to transitioning from perimenopause to menopause, or who cannot tolerate the hormone levels of birth control pills, might be better served by HRT. Women who take birth control pills for perimenopause can then switch to HRT during or after menopause, if they choose to do so.

## Low-Dose Birth Control Pills

Birth control pills have come a long way since their debut in the early 1960s. Today's version of "the Pill" contains just a fraction of the hormones of earlier versions, making it safer and less likely to produce side effects. Birth control pills reduce the symptoms of perimenopause by taking over control of ovulation. This stabilizes your body's hormone levels and restores regularity to your periods, which usually ends perimenopause and PMS symptoms (low-dose birth control pills are also the treatment of choice for PMS that fails to respond to lifestyle changes).

The type of birth control pill most commonly prescribed for perimenopause symptoms is *low-dose* and *monophasic*—it delivers the same levels of estrogen and progesterone throughout the month. You can continue taking birth control pills until it's likely that you've entered menopause, generally around age 52 or 53. It might be difficult for you to know when you've made this transition, however, because the birth control pill's infusion of hormones sustains the menstrual cycle and also suppresses

### Wise Up

**Low-dose** birth control pills contain lower doses of hormones than standard birth control pills. **Monophasic** birth control pills contain the same levels of estrogen and progesterone in each pill, unlike other birth control pills that contain varying levels of hormones for different weeks of the menstrual cycle.

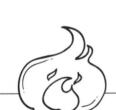

### Hot Flash!

Smoking and birth control pills do not mix! Numerous studies have shown that women who smoke face a significantly increased risk of blood clots, which can result in heart attack or a stroke.

symptoms such as hot flashes that might otherwise suggest that you've entered menopause. Some doctors suggest that women stop taking birth control pills for a few months to see whether they menstruate without them; other doctors recommend transitioning to HRT, if that's the woman's choice.

However, some women can't tolerate the birth control pill. They experience a wide range of side effects that resemble PMS. Other women shouldn't take birth control pills because of existing health conditions such as high blood pressure, heart disease, or liver disease, or because they smoke. Although at one time there was concern that birth control pills increased a woman's chance of getting breast cancer, numerous studies have concluded that this is not the case. In fact, it appears that the birth control pill can reduce the risk for several kinds of cancer, including ovarian, endometrial (uterine), and colorectal cancers. Birth control pills also reduce the risk of pelvic inflammatory disease (PID), osteoporosis, and noncancerous ovarian cysts. And, of course, birth control pills offer protection against unplanned pregnancy.

## Hormone Replacement Therapy (HRT)

Women who can't or don't want to use birth control pills sometimes get relief from the same kind of hormone replacement therapy (HRT) used during and after menopause. HRT is less effective than the birth control pill because the hormone levels are much lower. HRT does not affect ovulation, so some perimenopausal and PMS symptoms may continue as your body's natural hormone levels continue fluctuating. In addition, there is no birth control protection with HRT, so a woman might still become pregnant if she is ovulating.

# How Long Perimenopause Lasts

As we've said, perimenopause can last as long as 15 years, although most women move through it and into menopause within 3 to 6 years. When women and doctors in earlier decades perceived menopause to be a 15-year or longer event, what they were observing was actually perimenopause. Most women for whom perimenopause is a more extended experience have a few noticeable but not significant symptoms early on that let them know they are in perimenopause. The most disruptive symptoms are likely (although not guaranteed) to happen closer to menopause.

## The Possibility of Pregnancy

Although your body is preparing for menopause, it remains fertile. Your ovaries continue to produce viable eggs, if they have been doing so all along. If you've delayed pregnancy and now want to have a baby before menopause, this is good news. If you think that your body's signals mean you can forgo contraception, you could be in for some surprising news and a new family member.

Doctors generally consider a woman to be fertile until she has gone a full year (12 consecutive months) without a period. If your periods are irregular, or even if you miss several in a row, you could still be ovulating. In fact, if you are sexually active and miss a period or two, you might want to do a home pregnancy test or see your healthcare provider, just to be sure that perimenopause, not pregnancy, has altered your cycles.

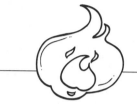

**Hot Flash!**

You can still become pregnant during perimenopause. If you want to conceive, talk with your healthcare provider about ways to optimize your chances. If you don't want to conceive, use a reliable birth control method.

## Menopause: The Calm After the Storm

After an erratic and often wild ride through perimenopause, many women find menopause to be a comparatively quiet and easy transition. Hormone swings during perimenopause are typically more extreme and rapid than they are during menopause, although as with menopause, some women experience few or no symptoms from them. Even as hormone levels fluctuate during menopause, they are diminishing.

## Self-Care During Perimenopause

Even in our equality-oriented modern times, most women spend much of their adult lives in the role of a caregiver. They might raise children or work in jobs that put them in the position of taking care of the needs of others. This becomes our orientation, and often we overlook the need to take care of ourselves. As the saying goes, you can't give from an empty cup. Perimenopause is a strong and persistent reminder that you need to pay attention to yourself as well. Treat yourself to an occasional evening alone. Visit a favorite bookstore, see a movie, or get a massage. A brisk walk every day will help you sleep better at night. For many women, the transitions of perimenopause and menopause take place when their children are grown enough to care for themselves or even move out, when their own jobs and careers are settled, and when they finally have time to think about themselves again.

**Wise Up**

**Weight-bearing exercise** is moderate to intense physical activity, such as jogging, that puts pressure on your skeletal system. **Osteoporosis** is a potentially serious health condition in which the bones lose calcium, making them fragile and susceptible to fractures.

## Keeping Your Body Healthy

Regular exercise and good nutrition are important at any stage in life, but they are especially important as you approach menopause. *Weight-bearing exercise* is one of the best ways to keep your body's calcium levels high. This is important for reducing the risk of *osteoporosis,* a potentially painful and debilitating condition in which bones become weakened and fragile due to loss of calcium. Resistance training is another form of exercise that's good for bone strength.

Increasing the amount of calcium in your diet is important, too. This is because your body's ability to absorb calcium from the foods you eat diminishes as you grow older. Your body becomes less efficient at extracting and converting calcium into forms that keep bones strong. You get less use from what you eat, so you need to increase the amounts of calcium-rich foods in your diet to compensate. Some studies show that increased calcium reduces the symptoms of PMS as well.

## Staying Calm and Comfortable

If relaxation techniques such as meditation or yoga have not been a part of your life, perimenopause is the ideal time to add them. When hormonal swings make you irritable and less tolerant, it becomes more challenging to manage the usual stresses of your life. Sometimes a caring partner or friend will gently point out to you that you're becoming quite snappy and short-tempered. Try to accept this observation in the spirit of kindness with which it was delivered. It's hard to see yourself and the changes that are taking place.

## The Least You Need to Know

➤ Perimenopause is not menopause. You are still fertile, still have periods, and still can become pregnant.

➤ Perimenopause can worsen PMS or bring it on for the first time.

➤ Birth control pills can provide relief from the discomfort of fluctuating hormones, as well as protection from unplanned pregnancy.

➤ Perimenopause can last from 3 to 15 years, although it averages from 3 to 6 years.

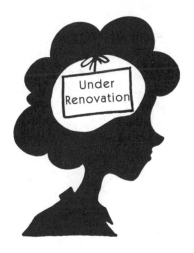

# Chapter 5

# Menopause and Your Body

---

## In This Chapter

➤ Understanding your reproductive system

➤ How your body functions before menopause

➤ How your body changes during menopause

➤ Is your body prepared for menopause? A self-quiz

➤ Go with the flow

---

Menopause brings about many changes in your body. In time, these changes will affect nearly every aspect of your life. To understand what happens during menopause, you need to know what organs and systems are involved and what their functions are before menopause. Although menopause ultimately affects all body parts and systems, it starts with those that play a role in reproduction.

These are the most obvious changes—menstruation becomes irregular and ultimately ceases, and your ability to bear children fades. These hormone-driven changes affect your sexuality and your perception of yourself as a woman. If you've chosen a child-free life, the changes taking place in your body may cause you to question your decision now that the element of choice is rapidly disappearing. If you've had children, you may experience sadness—or relief—about your diminishing fertility. And these inward changes have outward signs that you may welcome ... or resent.

# The Parts: Your Organs

The female reproductive organs represent a marvel in physiological engineering. They inhabit your lower abdomen, or pelvic region, and consist of the uterus, fallopian tubes, ovaries, cervix, and vagina.

The pear-shaped uterus, also called the womb, is a hollow muscular organ that rests just above the pubic bone with its narrow end pointed down and its broad, rounded top tipped slightly forward. Strong yet flexible ligaments anchor the uterus to the pelvis, giving it stability during pregnancy and childbirth. In its nonpregnant state, the uterus is about three inches long and weighs two to three ounces. During pregnancy, the uterus can expand to about 100 times its size. A thick, soft layer of tissue called the endometrium lines the interior of the uterus.

Attached to each side of the uterus by short tissue stems are the ovaries, the glands that produce the ova, or eggs, and the hormones responsible for the woman's reproductive cycle. Covering the ovary like tiny barnacles are thousands and thousands of follicles, tiny pockets that cradle undeveloped eggs. At birth, a baby girl has all the eggs she'll ever produce—about two million, evenly distributed between the two ovaries. Only a minute fraction of them, about 300, will mature to be released at ovulation throughout her lifetime. A mature ovum is barely visible to the naked eye, about the size of a needle's point. The rest of the eggs deteriorate, and their cellular material is reabsorbed into the body.

Extending from the top of the uterus are the fallopian tubes, one on each side. They curve downward and hang, open-ended, just above the ovaries. Surrounding each fallopian tube's opening are fimbriae, which look like fringe reaching toward the ovary. The fimbriae begin to gently undulate at ovulation, drawing the released ovum into the fallopian tube to begin its journey to the uterus. At the base of the uterus is the cervix, a muscular cuff of tissue that serves as the passageway between the uterus and the channel leading outside the body, the vagina.

*The female reproductive organs.*

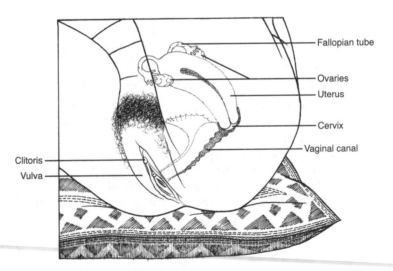

Fallopian tube

Ovaries

Uterus

Cervix

Vaginal canal

Clitoris

Vulva

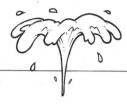

### Wellspring

Ancient physicians had many misperceptions about the organs of the female reproductive system. Greek and Roman physicians in the fourth century believed that the uterus wandered freely about in the woman's body, returning to its rightful position only when necessary (apparently for sex, pregnancy, and childbirth). The Greek physician Galen (130–200) taught his students that a woman's body was just like a man's except turned outside in. These perceptions persisted for many centuries, until scientific approaches to the human body revealed its internal secrets.

# The Messengers: Your Hormones

*Hormones* are chemical substances that regulate hundreds of specific body functions from metabolism (insulin) to reproduction (estrogens, progesterone, androgens). Your body produces hormones in structures called *glands,* which collectively comprise the *endocrine system.*

Your ovaries produce the hormones primarily responsible for menstruation and menopause—estrogen, progesterone, and testosterone. (Yes, your female body has small amounts of male hormones, just as male bodies have small amounts of female hormones.) Other hormones that play a role in the reproductive cycle are the follicle-stimulating hormone (FSH) and luteinizing hormone (LH), both produced by the pituitary gland, and androgens, produced by the adrenal glands. The adrenal glands, located along the tops of the kidneys, also produce small amounts of estrogen.

### Wise Up

**Hormones** are chemical messengers your body produces that stimulate or initiate certain events or actions. **Glands** are the structures within the body that produce hormones. The **endocrine system** is the network of your body's glands and hormones.

*The female endocrine system.*

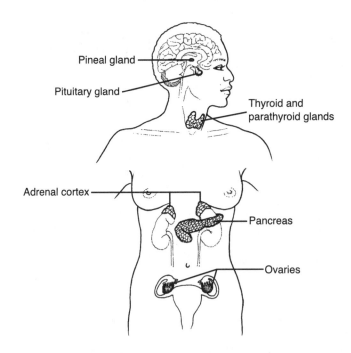

Pineal gland

Pituitary gland

Thyroid and parathyroid glands

Adrenal cortex

Pancreas

Ovaries

# The Mother Hormone: Estrogen

You might think of estrogen as the mother hormone. Produced primarily by the ovaries and to a limited extent by fat cells, estrogen is responsible for most of what we associate with womanhood: secondary sex characteristics, ovulation and menstruation, and implantation of the embryo to begin pregnancy. It also appears to have a nurturing role outside its participation in the reproductive cycle. Estrogen seems to help in healing wounds, maintaining bone strength, protecting a woman's heart and circulatory system from disease by raising "good" cholesterol and lowering "bad" cholesterol, and reducing the risk of certain cancers, as well as Alzheimer's disease. With menopause, estrogen production drops to less than a third of what it was during childbearing years.

# Preparing for Pregnancy: Progesterone

Progesterone's primary role is to prepare the body for pregnancy. Before pregnancy, the ovaries produce progesterone following ovulation to ready the uterus for conception, as well as to thin and neutralize the cervical mucus to create a more hospitable environment for sperm. During pregnancy, the placenta produces progesterone to keep the placenta functioning properly. With menopause, progesterone production drops to a small percentage of what it was during childbearing years.

## *Not Just for Men: Testosterone*

Testosterone, an androgen, influences a woman's sex drive. A woman's body produces and needs only a very small amount of testosterone. However, the decrease in testosterone level following menopause appears responsible for such undesirable effects as reduced sex drive, fatigue, and continued hot flashes. A woman's adrenal glands and ovaries both produce testosterone, although which produces the greater amount is not consistent. Some women who have their ovaries removed experience rapid and dramatic effects from suddenly lowered testosterone levels, while others barely notice the changes. With menopause, a woman's body generally produces about half the testosterone it did during childbearing years.

# Your Reproductive Cycle Before Menopause

At puberty, which is usually between ages 10 and 13 in American girls, hormone production kicks into high gear. The pituitary gland and the ovaries both start churning out the chemicals that will initiate the monthly cycle of menstruation. This cycle is a precise and complex choreography of events that will repeat every 26 to 35 days, except during pregnancy, for the next 40 to 45 years. To start the cycle, the pituitary gland releases FSH. FSH stimulates the ovary's follicles to ripen several ova. As it does so, the ovaries increase their output of estrogen, which causes the endometrium (lining of the uterus) to thicken and increase its blood supply in readiness for pregnancy.

About 14 days later, estrogen reaches a level that triggers the pituitary gland to release LH. LH serves as the chemical messenger telling the ovary's follicle to discharge its now-mature cargo, the ripened egg. The ovary carries out this mission with an explosive action somewhat like a sneeze, which sends the ovum out onto the ovary's surface. Once empty, the follicle produces progesterone. Progesterone turns the endometrium into a welcoming and nourishing environment for a prospective embryo.

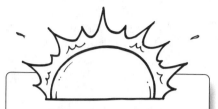

**Embracing Change**

A recent nationally representative survey of 1,000 women revealed that many of them didn't understand the role of hormones in menopause. While a third of them knew that estrogen had some involvement, only 8 percent knew that progesterone also was involved. This lack of knowledge was the reason nearly half of the women surveyed opted not to use HRT during and after menopause.

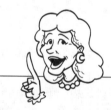

**Wise Woman's Wisdom**

"It seems necessary to completely shed the old skin before the new, brighter, stronger, more beautiful one can emerge ... I never thought I'd be getting a life lesson from a snake!"

—Julie Ridge

In the meantime, the fallopian tube's fimbriae gently pull the ovum in and send it on its way to the uterus. If conception is to take place, it usually does so in the fallopian tube. The fertilized egg continues to develop as it proceeds up the fallopian tube and into the uterus. By the time it arrives, it has reached the embryo stage. It implants itself into the blood-rich endometrium, and although the woman doesn't yet know it, pregnancy is underway. Implantation stimulates the follicle to continue producing progesterone, which maintains the environment the embryo needs to survive and grow.

If the egg is not fertilized, the follicle stops progesterone production. Without progesterone to support it, the endometrium sloughs away from the walls of the uterus. The egg mingles with the residual, and all of this material leaves the body through the vagina as menstrual discharge. It's been about three weeks since the pituitary gland released its surge of FSH, and in five to seven days—the duration of the menstrual period—it'll be time to do it all over again.

# What Happens Inside Your Body *During* Menopause

Although we tend to think of menopause in terms of the hormonal changes that take place, it's actually the deterioration of eggs that sets the entire process in motion. A woman's eggs begin deteriorating even before she is born and continue to do so throughout her life, but the effects don't become noticeable until the approach of menopause when finally so few eggs remain that hormone production is affected.

## *Hormone Heaven or Hell?*

The first clue that you're at menopause's doorstep is elevated FSH levels. FSH, the follicle-stimulating hormone, initiates the menstrual cycle by signaling the ovary's follicles to ripen an ovum. When the expected response fails to happen, there's a pause in the cycle. The pituitary gland sends more FSH, attempting to push the ovaries into action. During all this, estrogen levels remain low because the ovary has not received the signal to increase estrogen production. In fact, the cycle remains paused because none of the usual events are occurring. Periods become irregular, and unless the follicle finally responds by ripening and releasing an egg, the suspension becomes permanent. Your FSH level remains elevated, and your estrogen level drops.

While this is happening, your body is still expecting its surge of estrogen. When it doesn't get it, your body sometimes acts in strange and not fully understood ways. Estrogen seems to have some role in how the body regulates heat. When estrogen levels drop off, this regulatory process short-circuits somehow (no one really understands the precise reason or mechanism). It misinterprets the body's temperature as being too hot and floods the blood vessels near the skin in an effort to dissipate heat. The result is a rapid and intense flushing often followed by profuse sweating, as though you had just raced around the block. Because you're not really overheated, however, your body releases too much heat and often compensates by causing you to chill.

There are various approaches to reducing hot flashes, from HRT to acupuncture and biofeedback. Chapter 12, "Hot Flashes, Thinning Hair, and What's Happening *Down There,*" discusses relief and treatment options.

## This Is Your Brain at Menopause

Some evidence indicates that the hormonal changes of perimenopause and menopause affect the brain's chemistry and functions. This might explain why estrogen seems to reduce the risk of Alzheimer's disease. Some studies suggest that estrogen acts as an antioxidant to protect brain cells from being damaged by metabolic waste. When estrogen drops off after menopause, this protection diminishes, possibly contributing to loss of memory and cognitive ability (critical thinking). There are more questions than answers in this area, and much research is ongoing in an attempt to better understand the effects of hormones and the changes in them brought about through menopause.

## Biochemical Changes

Other biochemical changes take place in your body during and following menopause as well. Unfortunately, most of them seem to have detrimental effects unless you take actions to counter them. Bones can lose calcium, leading to osteoporosis, and arteries accumulate plaque, leading to heart disease (including high blood pressure and stroke). Metabolism slows, and your body's sensitivity to insulin decreases. Again, there are more questions than answers about what happens and why. Many risks are related to genetics, ethnicity, and other factors.

**Embracing Change**

If exercise is beginning to sound like a miracle cure for all that disturbs you about menopause, that's because exercise provides so many benefits. Not only does it help you maintain cardiovascular health and control your weight, but it also increases blood flow to the skin, reducing wrinkles and improving elasticity. And you feel better overall when you work your body a bit!

## Physical Changes

Nearly every part of a woman's body experiences physical changes as a result of menopause. Some are fairly obvious and immediate, such as the end of menstruation, thinning hair, and drier skin. Body fat proportions shift, with more fat settling around the hips and thighs (just what we need). In addition, the pelvis tends to widen as the shoulders narrow. Hair becomes thinner and grayer, and skin begins to fit less snugly.

Other changes are more subtle. By the time a woman is in her mid-40s, she is beginning to become shorter as a result of decreasing bone mass. About a third of all women will develop osteoporosis by the time they complete menopause, and they may lose up to 30 percent of their bone mass. Some studies show that starting at around age 35, women can lose 1 percent of bone mass per year. This might not sound like much, but it's a significant amount. Weight-bearing exercise and medications can stop and even somewhat reverse this loss.

# Is Your Body Prepared for Menopause?

That menopause is inevitable or imminent doesn't necessarily mean that your body is ready for it. Many of us cruise through life without giving too much thought to health and fitness. Hormones and busy lives seem to keep us fairly on track. But as both begin to slow down, less-than-healthful habits become more obvious.

## *Habitit, Habitat: A Self-Quiz*

How ready is your body for menopause? Take this short quiz to find out! Select the answer that best represents your situation.

1. When hunger overcomes you in the middle of the afternoon, you …
    a. Reach for that emergency chocolate bar in the back of your desk drawer.
    b. Nibble on the pretzels you didn't eat for lunch.
    c. Walk down to the deli on the corner and buy an apple.

2. Today's exercise is likely to be …
    a. Racing for the elevator.
    b. Walking from the back of the parking lot.
    c. Aerobic dance class at noon.

3. The food group from which you consume the most is …
    a. Caffeine and chocolate.
    b. Dairy products and meats.
    c. Vegetables and fruits.

4. You know you had a good night's sleep when …
    a. You only hit the alarm's snooze button twice.
    b. You come to life in the shower before you've had your morning coffee.
    c. You get out of bed just before the alarm goes off, feeling invigorated and eager to start the day.

5. If you had an unexpected afternoon free from your regular activities, you would …

   a. Catch up on the soaps.

   b. Take a nap.

   c. Take a brisk walk or bicycle ride.

6. Your favorite way to relax after a hectic and stressful day is to …

   a. Collapse on the couch with a glass of wine and the TV guide.

   b. Brew a cup of herbal tea and sit outside to drink it.

   c. Take a warm shower or bath, and then meditate or do yoga.

7. What you know about menopause you learned …

   a. From the stories your mother and grandmother told when they didn't know you were listening.

   b. By talking to your friends who have already gone through it.

   c. By reading and researching as much material as you could get your hands on.

If you have five or more Cs, treat yourself to a bowl of fresh strawberries and a walk through the park. Your lifestyle habits are fairly healthful. If you have five or more Bs, you might want to rethink some of your routines. Your lifestyle habits could use some improvement. If you have five or more As, your body is going to kick and fight all the way through menopause! Finish reading this book, and then sit down and write out a plan for using this life transition to make significant lifestyle changes.

## Nurturing Good Nutrition and Lifestyle Habits

In Chapter 4, "Perimenopause: Approaching Menopause," we started talking about the importance of good nutrition and regular exercise. We can't emphasize this enough. As you grow older, your metabolism slows. This is not necessarily a function of menopause, because men experience it, too. But it does mean that you need to watch what you eat, and eat less. At age 40, your body requires about 150 fewer calories a day to meet its nutritional needs than it did at age 30. But most of us miss this subtle cue, and as a result look in the mirror one day to find ourselves a bit on the plump side. In fact, the typical American woman gains 15 to 20 pounds during perimenopause and menopause. Nutritious eating and regular exercise are the most effective ways to prevent this.

Other lifestyle habits become more significant with menopause as well, especially those that can lead to diseases for which risks normally increase with age. These include smoking and excessive drinking, which are linked to lung disease, liver disease, and various forms of cancer. If you smoke, give yourself the gift of better health and a longer life: Stop! There are no known health benefits from smoking and literally hundreds of potential health risks. Doctors today have a number of methods to make quitting easier and more likely a permanent change.

# Menopause: It's a Process, Not a Moment

Most women look at menopause as a determined period of time in their lives: two or three years, somewhere in their 50s. Yes, it's true that menopause does occupy time in your life. But it's not static or clearly defined, like a hallway. Rather, menopause is a dynamic, flowing process, more like a river. You can float along for the ride, kick and scream in resistance, or steer your own course—the choice is yours. Either option will carry you through, of course. The choice is not about your destination, but about your journey.

---

### The Least You Need to Know

➤ Hormones play a key role in the functions of your reproductive system before, during, and after menopause.

➤ The diminishing number of eggs your ovaries produce is what triggers menopause.

➤ The changes of menopause affect all of your body's systems in some way.

➤ Preparing your body for menopause can make the transition easier.

---

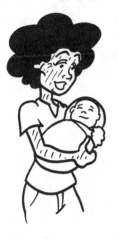

# Chapter 6

# Fertility, Midlife, and Menopause Babies

## In This Chapter

➤ What happens to fertility at age 40 and beyond

➤ The challenges of late-life pregnancy

➤ How medical technology can help women over age 40 who want to become pregnant

➤ How to cope with an unplanned "menopause baby"

While it might seem odd to have a chapter on fertility and pregnancy in a book about menopause, these topics are very relevant for women now facing closure of their fertile years.

Many women choose to delay starting a family. They may first want to complete their educations and establish their careers, or perhaps they just aren't ready for parenthood. Although a woman's most fertile years are from her late teens to her mid-30s, this seems like a comfortably long period of time—long enough, in fact, to lull us into believing that we still have all the time in the world to have children. After all, women have been having babies late in life forever—those often surprising "menopause babies." And with regular reports in the news of women in their 50s giving birth with the aid of medical technology, we've come to expect that we can have what we want, when we want it. But, even with technology, can we really fool Mother Nature?

# When Your 40th Birthday Wish Is for a Baby

Some women are startled when they realize that they're about to turn 40 and their time to have a baby is running out. They may have consciously chosen not to become pregnant or have not yet found the partner with whom they want to share such an important event and responsibility. And some are surprised and dismayed to discover that they may no longer have a choice to make.

# Are You Still Fertile at 40?

Most women who were fertile in their 20s and 30s are still fertile in their forties. Those who have been using birth control may not have a sense of their fertility until they begin trying to become pregnant. While about 90 percent of couples in their 20s who want to conceive will do so within a year, only about 50 percent of those in their 40s will become pregnant. After age 45, the percentage drops even lower, to about 10 percent. This doesn't rule out pregnancy by any means, as many women have unexpectedly discovered when the periods they've missed are due to pregnancy rather than menopause. But it does mean that becoming pregnant might take longer.

## All About Eggs

Your eggs begin to develop long before you're born, about three or four months after conception. By birth, they have already begun to deteriorate. And by the time you hit age 40, the eggs you have left are in less than ideal condition. The cell wall of a released egg might be stiffer and more difficult for a sperm cell to penetrate. Or, they might be more fragile than normal, so the egg falls apart before fertilization can take place. This doesn't mean that your eggs aren't any good, but it does mean that they may need close to ideal circumstances for fertilization to take place.

**Wise Up**

**Subfertility** is the natural reduction in fertility that occurs as a result of aging. **Infertility** is the situation of having tried for a year without success to conceive. **Assisted reproductive technology** (**ART**) is a group of high-tech procedures that produce conception without sexual intercourse.

## Subfertile Is Not Infertile

A woman's fertility peaks when she is in her early to mid-20s. By the time you reach your late 30s, you're about 30 percent less fertile than you were 10 years earlier. Although you still produce viable eggs, you might ovulate less regularly so it is more difficult for you to become pregnant. Doctors call this *subfertility*, and it is a natural aspect of growing older. *Infertility*, on the other hand, occurs when a year of trying to conceive has not produced a pregnancy. While aging is the primary cause of subfertility, there are many potential causes for infertility. Subfertility often responds well to relatively noninvasive medical assistance such as hormone treatment, while infertility may require advanced intervention such as *assisted reproductive technology (ART)*.

# Becoming Pregnant at Midlife

Even if later pregnancy has always been your plan, it's not easy to become a mother when all your friends are sending their children off to college or even becoming grandmothers already. Pregnancy at any age heralds a major life change, of course. You are about to become responsible for another life and to dedicate the next 20 years or so of your life to meeting his or her needs. This will keep you busy, no matter what your age.

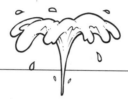

### Wellspring

Down's syndrome is a chromosomal disorder that results in variable physical and mental disabilities. While about 1 in every 600 to 800 infants born overall has Down's syndrome, the risk is related to the mother's age and takes dramatic leaps at ages 35 and 45. Although researchers know that Down's syndrome occurs when there is an extra chromosome, they don't yet understand where it comes from. Because the likelihood of having a baby with Down's syndrome increases with the mother's age, most researchers believe that the defect originates in the egg. Tests such as chorionic villus sampling and amniocentesis can obtain cells from the fetus that then undergo chromosome analysis. Although these tests can determine whether Down's syndrome exists, they cannot assess the degree of disability.

## *The Lowdown on Midlife Motherhood*

Some risks with late-life pregnancy are far less common in younger women. Older moms are more likely to conceive twins or triplets than are their younger counterparts, and they have an increased risk for the baby to have certain disorders such as Down's syndrome (see the previous Wellspring sidebar) or spina bifida (a condition in which bone and muscle tissue fail to enclose the spinal cord). Older women are also more likely to have complications during pregnancy, such as gestational diabetes or hypertension, as well as complications during delivery that require a Caesarean (surgical) delivery.

But there are advantages to late-life pregnancy, too. You are likely more mature, balanced, and realistic at age 40 than you were at age 25. As a result, you're likely to be more patient, dedicated, and reasonable with your child. This isn't to say that you'll have any easier time of it, just that your attitudes and expectations are different.

## The Physical Considerations of Pregnancy

Pregnancy at any age is a tremendous physical challenge for your body. Although it may seem like it takes a long time for you to "show," the developing fetus actually grows rapidly. It draws all the nutrients it needs to support its growth from you, even to the point of depleting your body of the nutrients it needs. For this reason, it's essential to eat nutritiously as well as take a prenatal vitamin supplement that is formulated to give you the additional support your body needs.

Your body changes in many ways during pregnancy, especially toward the end as it prepares for birth. Your uterus might expand to 100 times its prepregnancy size (or more, if you're carrying multiple babies). For the first time in your life, you can actually see what the inside of your belly button looks like because it appears to be turned nearly inside-out by the eighth or ninth month of pregnancy. Of course, you lose sight of your feet at about the same time—unless you're sitting with them propped up, which you should do as often as possible. Your breasts may shoot from a B cup to a D cup or larger as they prepare to nourish your baby following birth. And as your due date approaches, the ligaments in your pelvis (as well as in other parts of your body) begin to soften in preparation for the stretching they'll need to do to let the baby out.

**Embracing Change**

If you're planning to become pregnant, talk with your health-care provider about beginning a prenatal vitamin regimen. This will provide your body with additional folic acid and other nutritional supplements that optimize your health and reduce the risk of certain kinds of birth defects.

## The Emotional Considerations of Pregnancy

There are two dimensions to the emotional side of pregnancy. One is primarily hormonal. If you got weepy and unpredictable every month before your period, brace yourself for a wild ride on the emotional roller coaster. During pregnancy, your body produces dozens of hormones not present at any other time. These chemical messengers stay quite busy managing the process of pregnancy, assuring that every little thing functions just as it should. They go about this mission with a single-minded zeal, disrupting and realigning nearly every system in your body to fulfill their efforts. As a result, you can feel ecstatically euphoric, yet 10 minutes later burst into tears. You may cry at television commercials, magazine pictures, and songs on the radio. Although it's sometimes hard to maintain perspective, try to go with the flow.

All those little hormone messengers will pack their bags and hustle away, figuratively speaking, once their role concludes.

The other dimension of your emotions during pregnancy is more related to the stress and anxiety you might feel about being pregnant, giving birth, and raising a child. These feelings, too, are normal. After all, this is a major life event—you should expect to worry just a little bit about what effects this is going to have.

If worries and fears occupy most of your waking thoughts and infiltrate your dreams, however, discuss them with your healthcare provider. Often, just being able to confront your anxieties can put them into perspective.

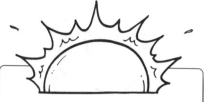

**Embracing Change**

Strive to surround yourself with positive encouragement and support during pregnancy. As much as possible, turn a deaf ear to those who feel compelled to share their horror stories. Every woman's experience with pregnancy and delivery is unique.

## Your Support Network

It's important to have a circle of family and friends to whom you can turn for support with everything from household chores to talking about your concerns. These should be caring individuals who can comfort you when you need a shoulder to cry on as well as share a laugh with you. They should support your decision to become pregnant at your oh-so-old age and should welcome the changes your decision is bringing into your life. Some people can't do this, and you don't need their skepticism. Many communities have support groups for midlife moms, difficult pregnancies, and other needs.

# Exploring High-Tech Possibilities

While half of women over age 40 who choose to become pregnant do so with little effort or complications, half of them don't. Most doctors don't become concerned about fertility issues until you've tried to get pregnant for a year without success, or if you're over age 45. In these situations, you might need a boost from medical technology. Because this is a highly specialized area of medicine, your regular healthcare provider will refer you to a fertility specialist for further evaluation and treatment.

## What You Should Know About Fertility Drugs

Fertility drugs are hormones that stimulate ovulation. Because most fertility problems in women are related to egg production and ovulation, these drugs are often the first course of treatment (following evaluation to determine whether there are other

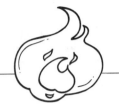

physical problems, such as blocked fallopian tubes). The drug the fertility specialist chooses to use depends on many factors, and your doctor may prescribe a combination of drugs if there are multiple components to your ovulatory problem.

There are two significant risks associated with fertility drugs: ovarian hyperstimulation syndrome (OHSS), a medical condition in which potentially dangerous levels of fluid accumulate in the woman's body, and multiple-gestation pregnancy, in which a woman may conceive twins, triplets, or higher multiples.

OHSS can be a very serious medical condition if the retained fluid begins to put pressure on vital organs such as the lungs, heart, and liver. It may require medical intervention and sometimes hospitalization. OHSS occurs in 1 to 5 percent of drug-induced ovulation and is not predictable. Multiple-gestation pregnancy occurs in about 20 percent of women who use fertility drugs, a rate that is 10 to 20 times greater than with an unassisted pregnancy. This is because fertility drugs stimulate the ovaries to ripen and release more ova. Your doctor can minimize the risk of multiple-gestation pregnancy by carefully monitoring both the drug's dosage and its effects. If it appears that you've released too many eggs, your doctor can let you know and recommend that you not try to conceive on that cycle.

## Intrauterine Insemination (IUI): Hit the Spot

Intrauterine insemination (IUI) involves placing a specially concentrated and treated sperm collection directly into the uterus at ovulation. This bypasses the most hazardous part of the sperm's journey, giving a much-improved chance of fertilization. The procedure is done in the fertility specialist's office and usually doesn't hurt, although some women experience mild cramping afterward. IUI is usually done in conjunction with fertility drug treatment to assure that the woman produces a viable egg at ovulation.

## The ART of Conception: IVF, GIFT, and ZIFT

More extensive fertility treatments are called assisted reproductive technology (ART). They include in vitro fertilization (IVF), gamete intrafallopian transfer (GIFT), and zygote intrafallopian transfer (ZIFT). These procedures are more extensive than fertility drug treatment or IUI, and they are invasive because they involve retrieving eggs from the woman, which is done under intravenous sedation or a general anesthetic. GIFT and ZIFT also involve laparoscopic surgery to transfer the fertilized eggs back into the woman.

The most commonly used ART is IVF, also known as the "test-tube baby" technique. In IVF, the fertility specialist removes eggs from the woman and fertilizes them with sperm from her partner (or a donor) in laboratory dish (not actually a test tube). If fertilization takes and embryos develop, the fertility specialist transfers the embryos into the uterus. Hopefully, one of the embryos will implant just as if it had arrived in the usual fashion via the fallopian tube. The possiblity of multiple gestation exists with this procedure. Drug therapy is used to assure consistent hormone levels to sustain the pregnancy after implantation.

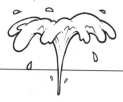

### Wellspring

An experiment in England in 1978 produced the world's first test-tube baby, Louise Brown. She was conceived through in vitro fertilization (IVF), a procedure in which the egg and sperm are united in a laboratory dish rather than within the fallopian tube. Since Louise's birth, more than 20,000 babies have been conceived through IVF in the United States alone, and thousands more have been conceived worldwide. Today, about one-third of IVFs result in births. The procedure is no longer experimental but is a staple of fertility treatment.

In GIFT, the fertility specialist retrieves several eggs while the woman is under a general anesthetic. The eggs are immediately added to a sperm sample (either her partner's or a donor's) and are placed into the woman's fallopian tube using laparoscopic surgery. In ZIFT, things start out as in IVF, with the eggs being fertilized in the lab. Then, as in GIFT, the fertilized eggs (called zygotes) are placed in the woman's fallopian tube through laparoscopic surgery.

## Considering Donor Egg or Surrogacy

Sometimes a woman's eggs have deteriorated to the point at which they cannot be fertilized. If this is the case, donor eggs are an option to consider. The procedure typically uses IVF, although it may sometimes use GIFT or ZIFT. The resulting child would not have your genetic material, but you would carry the pregnancy. For women who cannot sustain pregnancy, surrogacy might be an option. In this setting, the fertilized egg (usually yours, fertilized by your partner's sperm, although both sperm and egg could be supplied by donors) is transferred to a surrogate, who carries the pregnancy and gives birth to the baby on your behalf. There are many legal issues to consider with these options, however, so it is to your advantage to consult with an attorney who specializes in such matters before signing any contracts.

## What You Need to Know About Costs and Insurance

In a nutshell, fertility assistance is quite expensive and often is not covered by insurance. A resulting pregnancy usually is covered, however, except for surrogacy. It's possible to spend tens to hundreds of thousands of dollars on fertility treatments, with no guaranteed results.

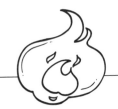

### Hot Flash!

Check the details of your health insurance before beginning medical care and treatment for infertility. Health plans differ according to their policies and practices. Some services may be covered if claims are submitted under certain codes but could be disallowed under other codes. Those that do offer coverage for some fertility services may require pre-approval or treatment from certain providers.

## Other Options: Adoption and Living Child-Free

If you want to raise a child that you can love as your own, adoption may be an option to consider. Although several recent high-profile situations have highlighted the potential problems of adoption, most adoptions that follow accepted guidelines go smoothly. If you're considering adoption, it's a good idea to consult with an attorney who specializes in this area for advice and suggestions.

If adoption doesn't appeal to you, or if you choose to live child-free, there are still plenty of ways to satisfy your desires to nurture and love a child. If you have nieces and nephews, "borrow" them once in a while. This gives you a chance to spend time with them and get to know them, and it gives their parents a chance to enjoy some time alone together without worrying about their kids. You could also volunteer at a local school or library, to read or assist with other activities, or enroll in a mentoring program.

## Just When You Thought It Was Safe ...

At the other end of the late-life pregnancy spectrum are the women in their late 40s or even early 50s who are stunned to learn that their periods have stopped not because of menopause, but because of pregnancy. Just as they were gearing up for—and even looking forward to—the next stage in the cycle of their lives and thought that they could no longer become pregnant, they're planning for a new family member.

Instead of meeting with the gynecologist to discuss HRT, they're scheduling eight months of appointments with the obstetrician.

Fertility is one of life's great mysteries. It doesn't seem quite fair that while some women who want to conceive later in life find that they no longer have the ability to do so, other women who don't want to become pregnant do. Although precise figures are difficult to determine, late-life unexpected pregnancies are not that uncommon.

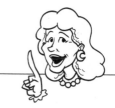

**Wise Woman's Wisdom**

"After 30, a body has a mind of its own."

—Bette Midler

## How Long Is Birth Control Necessary?

While the generally accepted guideline is that women remain fertile until a full year—12 consecutive months—have passed without having a period, women whose periods have become quite irregular may not fully transition beyond menopause within this timeline. The only sure way to determine that you're no longer fertile is to have your FSH levels tested over a period of a few months after you believe that you have completed menopause. If they remain elevated, you are no longer fertile. If they fluctuate, however, the possibility of pregnancy still exists, even though it's remote.

If you definitely do not want to become pregnant, you must use a reliable form of birth control until you can clearly and definitively establish that you've transitioned through menopause. For many women, this can be well into their 50s. A key advantage of taking birth control pills during this time, in fact, is that it prevents pregnancy at the same time it reduces the signs of menopause. Not all women can or want to take birth control pills, however. If you are among them, discuss your options with your healthcare provider. You might want to consider sterilization (either a tubal ligation for you or a vasectomy for your partner) to assure that you will not become pregnant.

## Accepting and Adapting to a Surprise Pregnancy

Unexpected late-life pregnancy can be quite a jolt. For some women, pregnancy presents a crisis of choice—do you keep or terminate? Age alone is not necessarily a reason to do either. Your health and other circumstances are more important than whether you're 20 or 40 years old. And how to handle an unplanned pregnancy is a deeply personal decision for any woman, regardless of age. Your choice should reflect reasons that are meaningful for you.

Many women who find themselves pregnant in midlife can enjoy a normal, healthy pregnancy and delivery. Because your age makes your pregnancy high-risk, as we discussed earlier in this chapter, you'll need to take extra precautions to assure your health and the health of your baby. Rally your support network—partner, siblings, other children, friends—for help. Having others you can turn to helps reduce the burden of responsibility that you may suddenly feel. Sure, you might find yourself confronting the terrible twos and the change of life at the same time, you might be the oldest room mother in kindergarten, and your friends might have grandchildren older than your child. But the unexpected has its ways of working out. You have the wisdom of age, the patience of experience, the humor of perspective, and the strength of love to offer your newest family member. No child, planned or not, can expect more than that.

## The Least You Need to Know

➤ Pregnancy is still possible until at least a full year (12 consecutive months) has passed since your last period.

➤ Medical technology can greatly enhance your chances of becoming pregnant after age 40.

➤ A woman over age 40 is a third less fertile than she was at age 25.

➤ Late-life pregnancy is not without its challenges and risks—or its joys.

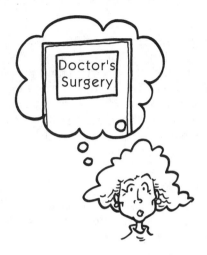

# Chapter 7

# Do You Need Your Uterus? Hysterectomies and Surgical Menopause

## In This Chapter

➤ The role of your uterus before and after menopause

➤ Reasons to consider having a hysterectomy

➤ Knowing the risks and the benefits

➤ The different surgical procedures for a hysterectomy

➤ What happens before, during, and after surgery

➤ Treatment options other than surgery

You do have to wonder: Why bother keeping your uterus after menopause if all that awaits you is trouble? Wouldn't it just make sense to take it out when you're not going to be using it anymore? While there are many reasons to consider surgical removal of your uterus, convenience isn't one of them. Like any medical treatment, surgery has risks. If you're considering a hysterectomy, you should be sure that the benefits outweigh the risks and that you understand both.

Just 20 years ago, hysterectomy was the most commonly performed surgery in the United States. There just weren't many options for problems such as persistent heavy bleeding and recalcitrant fibroids. Today, however, medical technology provides a number of alternatives to hysterectomy. Hysterectomy remains a successful treatment for many women, of course, and is the treatment of choice for conditions such as cancer. But it's worthwhile to evaluate all your choices before making your decision.

# Your Uterus and You

Your uterus has been a defining element of who you are since your birth. Although the ovaries really do most of the work as far as establishing a woman's female characteristics, the uterus is most noticeable. It bleeds every month. It carries an unborn child from conception to birth and then forcefully propels the child into the world to begin its own life. For many women, the uterus symbolizes the essence of womanliness. When you lose your uterus, you no longer menstruate or have the ability to become pregnant. For some women this is a relief, while others mourn the loss.

## Your Uterus Before Menopause

Before menopause, your uterus has a single mission: to incubate a baby. Each month, nudged into action by your body's hormone messengers, it dutifully prepares a nourishing and protective environment for a prospective resident. When there isn't one, it flushes away its preparations and then repeats the process. The uterus in its nonpregnant state is roughly about the size of your closed fist.

## Your Uterus After Menopause

After menopause, your uterus really has no role and gradually atrophies or shrinks. It loses both muscle and connective tissue. The endometrium thins to a membranelike lining. If you've had uterine fibroids (see the section "Fibroids" later in this chapter), they also shrink following menopause. Hormone replacement therapy (HRT) that includes both estrogen and progesterone reduces the degree of atrophy that takes place.

Some women experience a relaxing of the ligaments that hold the uterus in place. This can cause a condition called prolapse, in which the uterus pushes the cervix down into the vagina. Prolapse is painless for most women, although some women experience low back discomfort. Prolapse can become a medical problem if the sagging uterus puts enough pressure on pelvic structures to interfere with urination. Special exercises to strengthen and tighten the pelvic muscles, called Kegel exercises (named after the gynecologist who developed them), can often reduce or prevent prolapse before it occurs. After prolapse occurs, some women get temporary relief from a device called a pessary that is inserted into the vagina to hold pressure against the cervix. However, only surgery can permanently repair the condition.

## Your Cervix, Fallopian Tubes, and Ovaries

Once hormonal stimulation stops, the rest of your reproductive organs slowly atrophy as well. This does not generally create any health problems, although the cervix and ovaries are potential sites for cancer to develop. There's more on this a little later in this chapter.

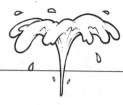

**Wellspring**

Although many organs in the human body are known by names closely related to the original Greek or Latin terms that first described them, it's unusual for one organ to retain both origins in different uses. The uterus takes its name from the Latin word *udero*, which means "abdomen." Yet most medical procedures use the Greek root word, *hystera*, which means "womb." And yes, it's true that *hysterectomy* and *hysteria* share common ancestry. This stems from the erroneous conclusion of ancient physicians that extreme emotions in women arose from the uterus.

# Why Your Doctor Might Recommend Hysterectomy

Nearly 600,000 American women have *hysterectomies* each year. Hysterectomy is often recommended to treat the following conditions:

➤ Cancer of the uterus (endometrial cancer) and sometimes of the cervix or ovaries

➤ Uterine fibroids (noncancerous tumors), especially those that grow rapidly, cause persistent bleeding and pain, or fail to respond to more conservative treatment

➤ Persistent bleeding that fails to respond to other treatment

➤ Endometriosis (uterine tissue that grows outside the uterus) that fails to respond to other treatment

➤ Uterine prolapse, when it causes problems with urination or bowel movements

More than two thirds of hysterectomies are performed to treat uterine fibroids, noncancerous tumors that often cause pain and bleeding. The other one third of them are done to treat the conditions for which removing the uterus is a treatment option. Except when done to treat some cancers, hysterectomy is nearly always an *elective surgery*, so you have time to consider other options and

**Wise Up**

A **hysterectomy** is the surgical removal of the uterus. An **elective surgery** is one that is necessary but not urgent.

67

obtain a second opinion if you wish (more on this a bit later).

## Cancer and Other Tumors

Menopause does not increase your risk of getting cancer—not breast, uterine, cervical, or ovarian cancer. Nearly all forms of cancer are more common with age, however, giving the impression that there is a correlation between menopause and "female" cancers. There are concerns that certain HRT approaches may increase the risk for uterine cancer, especially when treatment uses estrogen only. For a discussion of the risks and benefits of HRT, see Chapter 14, "What Is Hormone Replacement Therapy (HRT)?"

Surgery is the treatment of choice for most cancers, including those involving the female reproductive organs. A hysterectomy may be recommended for cancer of the uterus and the cervix. The uterus is also often removed, along with the ovaries and fallopian tubes, to treat ovarian cancer. When the cancer is detected and treated early in its development, the treatment success rate is very high. Depending on the stage and kind of cancer, the doctor might recommend follow-up treatment with chemotherapy or radiation therapy.

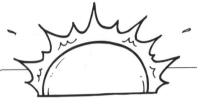

**Embracing Change**

Most women fear breast cancer, but lung cancer actually claims more lives. The majority of lung cancer is a direct result of cigarette smoking. To give yourself the best defense against cancer, get regular checkups that include a breast exam, a pelvic exam, and a Pap smear. And if you smoke, quit!

## Fibroids

Fibroids, also called myomas or fibromyomas, are noncancerous tumors made of muscle and connective tissue that grow from the wall of the uterus. Some grow rapidly and become quite large, while others grow slowly and stay fairly small. By age 40, about two thirds of American women have fibroids, although more than half of them experience few or no symptoms. When fibroids do present symptoms, they generally cause bleeding and pain. Although doctors know that estrogen causes fibroids to grow, they don't know what actually causes fibroids to develop in the first place.

It is possible to become pregnant if you have fibroids, although the fibroids can interfere with implantation. This can result in increased risk for miscarriage, premature labor, and malpresentation during delivery (such as a breech presentation). If you know you have fibroids and you want to become pregnant, discuss your options with your doctor. You might want to first treat the fibroids to reduce the potential that they'll interfere with pregnancy.

Sometimes fibroids respond to less invasive treatment such as medication (contraceptives and hormones) and localized surgery, called myomectomy, which removes the fibroids but leaves the uterus. As often as not, however, these treatments are temporary and the fibroids return. A new procedure that might offer hope and relief to women who want to avoid hysterectomy but still get rid of their fibroids is uterine artery embolization. This procedure uses injected particles to block the blood supply to the fibroid, causing it to shrink or even disappear.

## Endometriosis

In endometriosis, fragments of endometrium (the lining of the uterus) appear outside the uterus. These fragments, called implants, can attach themselves to various tissues in the abdominal cavity and, on rare occasions, even migrate to other parts of the body. Because the implants are endometrial, they enlarge and then bleed with each menstrual period. Mild endometriosis can be annoying and uncomfortable, while severe endometriosis can cause infertility, scarring, and pain. Doctors don't know what causes endometriosis.

Treatments such as laser or laparoscopic surgery to remove implants are usually only partly successful at obtaining relief, although this is the treatment of choice for women who want to become pregnant. Sometimes birth control pills taken continuously for up to a year (instead of stopping for a week each month for menstruation) cause endometrial implants to shrink. For many women with severe endometriosis, however, total hysterectomy with bilateral salpingo-oophorectomy (removing the uterus, cervix, ovaries, and fallopian tubes) is the only way to cure the condition.

## "As Long as We're in There ..."

There is a tendency for surgeons to want to do whatever they can once they've made an incision. To a great extent, this is common sense and can be an effective preventive measure. Sometimes surgeons will clean up adhesions (tissues that are stuck together, usually from scarring from other surgeries or from infections). It's important to clearly understand what your surgeon intends to do once you're opened up on the operating table, and to know if there are any additional risks.

## What Really Needs to Come Out?

Sometimes the medical problem necessitating surgery defines what needs to come out. With cervical cancer, for example, the surgeon will probably want to remove all the reproductive organs, as well as nearby tissue and lymph glands. In other situations, however, you may have some choice in what comes out and what stays in. It's best to discuss your individual situation with your surgeon before you plan or schedule the surgery. If you're not sure what to do, get a second opinion.

# Tubes and Ovaries

Generally, there's no reason to remove your fallopian tubes and ovaries, a surgical procedure called a salpingo-oophorectomy (bilateral, if both sides are removed) unless they are damaged or diseased, especially before menopause. Your ovaries continue to function even if your uterus is removed, which gives you the benefits of the hormones they produce. The ovaries and the cervix are potential sites for cancer, which is one reason the gynecologist may recommend their removal along with the uterus in a hysterectomy performed after menopause. We discuss the different kinds of hysterectomies a little later in this chapter.

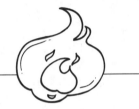

**Hot Flash!**

Medical treatment, including surgery, is always a matter of choice—*your* choice. Be sure that you fully understand your condition, all treatment options, and why your doctor is recommending surgery.

# Why Remove Your Appendix?

Some surgeons will remove your appendix, if you still have it, if you have an abdominal hysterectomy. Your doctor is especially likely to recommend this if you have chronic pelvic pain, since appendicitis is one potentially serious cause. The reasoning behind this is that your body has no use for your appendix, yet appendicitis can be a serious condition requiring emergency surgery. The rationale is that you might as well take it out while your belly is already open. To a degree, this makes good sense. There's no reason to have two surgeries if one can prevent the other.

However, during just a hysterectomy, there is no reason for the surgeon to cut your intestines. They're simply moved aside to give access to your uterus, and then they're replaced. Removing your appendix, which is a tiny pouchlike structure hanging from a corner of your colon (large intestine), involves cutting and repairing the intestine. The risk in this is that the bacteria naturally found within the intestine—and kept contained there by the intestinal walls—can escape into your abdominal cavity. This could cause an infection. With modern surgical techniques and preventive antibiotics, this doesn't happen often. Many surgeons believe it's far less risky to remove the appendix during another abdominal surgery rather than after it has become inflamed and infected, while others prefer not to intervene any more than is necessary. Talk to your doctor about your personal circumstances and needs.

# Understanding the Risks

Every surgery has risks. Some, such as infection and bleeding, are common to all surgeries. Others are specific to the kind of surgery being performed. General anesthesia—in which you're "put to sleep" using powerful drugs—also carries risks. It is important that you understand the risks of the surgery that your doctor is recommending. You should also have a clear understanding of any treatment options besides surgery and the consequences of choosing not to have the surgery.

## Informed Consent

*Informed consent* is a formal process by which your surgeon, and often the anesthesiologist, can give you complete and comprehensive information about the surgery you are about to have. This includes potential benefits as well as possible risks. Most hospitals require you to sign an informed consent form stating that you have received and understand this information. If you don't understand something about your condition or the planned surgery, ask for an explanation before you sign the form.

**Wise Up**

**Informed consent** is medical jargon for presenting you with full and complete information about the benefits and risks of the procedure your doctor recommends. Most hospitals require you to sign a form stating that these benefits and risks have been explained to you, and you understand and accept them.

## Getting a Second Opinion

A second opinion is always a good idea when considering elective surgery (and often with other treatments as well). Many people worry that their doctors will get angry or upset if they go to see another doctor, but most doctors encourage second opinions. A second opinion is not second-guessing your doctor. It's getting an examination from a different doctor, usually a specialist not connected to the first doctor in any way, to see if he or she concurs with the first doctor's diagnosis, assessment, and recommendation. Some insurance companies require a second opinion before authorizing coverage for an elective surgery.

# Hysterectomy: The Procedure Options

The surgeon can perform a hysterectomy in several ways. Often the preferred procedure depends on the problem being treated, although sometimes you can decide to have one instead of another.

## Abdominal Hysterectomy

In an abdominal hysterectomy, the surgeon makes a relatively long incision through the abdomen along the pubic hairline, or a vertical line between the umbilicus (belly button) and pubic bone. It's easy to reach in and remove the uterus, ovaries, and fallopian tubes all through this incision. There are also variations of the abdominal hysterectomy:

➤ A **subtotal hysterectomy** removes just the uterus.

➤ A **total hysterectomy** removes the uterus and the cervix.

➤ A **total hysterectomy with bilateral salpingo-oophorectomy** removes the uterus, the cervix, both ovaries, and both fallopian tubes.

➤ A **radical hysterectomy** removes the uterus, the cervix, the upper portion of the vagina, both ovaries and fallopian tubes, and surrounding lymph glands. It is typically used only to treat cervical cancer.

An abdominal hysterectomy is definitely major surgery. The surgeon cuts in-between major muscles and the abdominal wall to reach the uterus. There is a risk of damaging nerves and other tissues, and full recovery can take six to eight weeks.

## Vaginal Hysterectomy

A vaginal hysterectomy is the least invasive procedure for removing the uterus. The surgeon works through an incision inside the vagina, at the top along the cervix. This procedure is not always an option, though. A uterus filled with large fibroids, for example, usually cannot be removed through the small incision inside the vagina. The advantages of vaginal hysterectomy include less time in surgery, quicker recovery, and no external scar.

## Laparoscopically Assisted Vaginal Hysterectomy (LAVH)

In laparoscopically assisted vaginal hysterectomy (LAVH), the surgeon inserts special lighted instruments through small incisions in the abdomen to more easily remove organs such as the fallopian tubes and the ovaries, and sometimes scar tissue from previous surgeries or infections. Then the surgeon makes an incision from inside the vagina, as in a vaginal hysterectomy, and completes the surgery by removing what remains through this incision. The advantage of LAVH is that it is a less invasive procedure than an abdominal hysterectomy, yet it allows more surgeries to be done through the smaller vaginal incision.

# Preparing Your Body and Your Mind for Surgery

Because hysterectomy is seldom an emergency procedure, you'll have plenty of time to prepare your body and your mind for surgery. It's important to eat nutritiously so that your body has the resources it needs to heal and recover. It's common and natural to feel apprehensive, worried, or even fearful about surgery. You can calm and relax yourself with guided visualization techniques in which you envision your body opening itself to the surgery and healing itself afterward.

It's also often helpful to think about how you define your womanliness, and how having a hysterectomy might affect your sense of yourself as a woman. What do you perceive yourself to be losing? What can replace this loss? You might record your thoughts and concerns in a journal to help identify them and arrive at ways to resolve them. Your doctor or anesthesiologist can put you in touch with resources for learning guided imagery to help you envision a successful surgery and recovery. Many hospitals offer instruction in various self-healing techniques.

## What Happens Before Surgery

Most of the time, a hysterectomy requires a short stay in the hospital, generally one to three days. You can usually go to the hospital on the morning your surgery is scheduled. Many surgeons prefer to have the pubic region shaved. Some want a hospital technician to do this, while others are willing to let you do it yourself. Some surgeons prefer for their patients to receive an enema the morning before surgery, to clear the bowels. Again, some want this done at the hospital and others will let you do it at home. If you usually take medications, ask your doctor whether you should take them the day of your surgery.

## What to Expect After Surgery

Many women are up and walking—albeit slowly and carefully—the same evening after surgery, and certainly by the next morning. Post-operative pain may last for several days, although it dramatically improves with each passing day. Some women have difficulty urinating following surgery, particularly if a catheter was inserted during surgery. Gastrointestinal distress is also a common problem because bowel function is often slow to return. Moving around and walking are the best ways to help get your body functions back to normal.

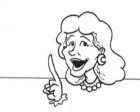

**Wise Woman's Wisdom**

"Happiness is good health and a bad memory."

—Ingrid Bergman

## When Will You Be Back to Normal?

How quickly you return to your normal activities depends on the kind of hysterectomy you have. With a LAVH or a vaginal hysterectomy, you could be back to your routine in two weeks. With an abdominal hysterectomy, you're likely to return to your usual activities in about six to eight weeks. Recovery is a very personal process that depends on numerous factors. It's important not to rush to return just for the sake of being back in your regular life events.

## Surgical or Induced Menopause

Surgical menopause, also called induced menopause, occurs when your ovaries are removed or damaged before you have completed menopause. Their sudden absence can be jarring to your body, and you may experience more intense menopausal changes

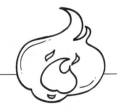

**Hot Flash!**

Regular GYN exams are important even after hysterectomy. If your cervix remains, you can still get cervical cancer. And the virus responsible for cervical cancer can also cause vaginal cancer.

than if you had transitioned through menopause naturally. Depending on your age and other health factors, your doctor may recommend HRT or other interventions. Chemotherapy, radiation therapy, and other events that permanently damage the ovaries can also produce induced menopause.

## Potential Complications

Whether vaginal or abdominal, a hysterectomy is major surgery. Most of the time, it goes well and women fully recover without any problems or complications. Occasionally, however, things don't go so smoothly. Every surgery carries risks of complications during and following the procedure, from unusual bleeding to infection. There also can be damage to bowel and urinary tract, as well as reactions to or complications resulting from the anesthesia. It's important to know what complications are possible so that you can report any signs of them to your doctor immediately.

# Alternatives to Hysterectomy

Except with cancer, a hysterectomy is seldom the first path of treatment that a doctor recommends or that you would want to follow. The conditions that ultimately may require a hysterectomy generally develop gradually, often over several years. The milder your symptoms, the less urgent the need for surgical treatment. Because surgery has risks and potential complications, you want to be sure that the positives outweigh the negatives before you sign on the dotted line.

## Watchful Waiting

When your symptoms are mild and your doctor has ruled out any problem needing immediate treatment, such as cancer or ectopic pregnancy, watchful waiting is often the best option. Some problems, such as excessive bleeding, can be temporary or self-limiting. Other problems may continue for months or years before they get to the point that they demand intervention. If your doctor is watchfully waiting with your condition, you'll probably have regular visits scheduled to check on your status. If any changes occur, your doctor will discuss potential treatment needs. Watchful waiting can be unsettling in a time when instant gratification is the norm, but often it's the least risky option when your condition could improve on its own or is likely to take a long time to worsen.

## *Natural and Complementary Therapies*

Sometimes natural or complementary therapies can help relieve your symptoms and discomfort. Herbs, acupuncture, meditation, and biofeedback are among the options that might help your condition. The chapters in Part 5, "Menopause Treatment *Au Naturel*," provide a thorough discussion of natural and complementary therapies.

## *HRT and Other Medical Approaches*

Hormone replacement therapy, birth control pills, and other medications can sometimes provide relief from symptoms such as heavy bleeding, cramping, and other discomfort. Sometimes these medical approaches give your body the respite it needs to heal itself. Other times they provide just temporary relief. The chapters in Part 4, "HRT or No HRT, That Is the Question," provide a comprehensive discussion of HRT.

---

### The Least You Need to Know

➤ Hysterectomy ends menstruation, fertility, and your ability to carry a pregnancy.

➤ Some women feel a sense of loss after a hysterectomy, as though they also lost a piece of their femininity. Although this is perfectly natural, there is no reason to feel that you are any less of a woman because you no longer have a uterus.

➤ Some women find that hysterectomy affects sexual function and pleasure; others do not.

➤ Some women feel an overwhelming sense of relief following hysterectomy. If they've struggled a long time with medical problems that the hysterectomy has eliminated, they often feel more alive and whole than they have for years.

➤ Hysterectomy doesn't necessarily hasten or cause menopause. As long as your ovaries remain, your body can continue producing hormones just as if you still had a uterus.

---

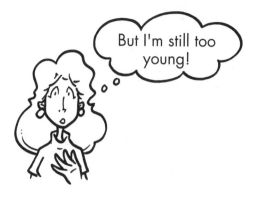

# Chapter 8

# Early Menopause

## In This Chapter

➤ Why menopause arrives early for some women

➤ The role of autoimmune disorders

➤ How family history influences the onset of menopause

➤ The effects of cigarette smoking on estrogen levels

➤ Coping with the emotions of early menopause

➤ The possibility of delaying early menopause

Most women experience the transition from fertility to nonfertility in midlife. For some women, however, the journey starts early—as much as 10 to 20 years ahead of schedule. Many factors influence the onset of menopause, no matter when it occurs. When your second spring arrives while the summer of your life is still in full bloom, it can bring with it a number of emotional and physical challenges.

For most women who experience it, early menopause comes as a shock. You may have put off having children until your career was settled or you felt ready to be a parent, and now suddenly the choice is no longer yours. Simply the new reality of living with the changes of menopause—of feeling old in a young body—can be tough to navigate and accept. Though sometimes the causes of early menopause are clear, they aren't always reversible. And more often than not, early menopause occurs for no apparent reason.

# What Is Early Menopause?

Typically a woman reaches menopause when she's in her early 50s, although the range of "normal" extends from the mid-40s to the early 60s. *Early menopause* takes place before the beginning of this range, when a woman is in her early 40s or younger. Sometimes a woman begins experiencing the signs of menopause extremely early, when she's in her 30s or even her 20s. This form of early menopause is called *premature menopause*.

Premature menopause is *not* the same as perimenopause (see Chapter 4, "Perimenopause: Approaching Menopause"). Perimenopause, the time (often years) of signs that herald the coming of menopause, often precedes premature menopause as well as normal menopause.

Premature menopause strikes during a woman's prime childbearing years. This is particularly distressing for women who have delayed getting pregnant yet want to have children, especially if they had no inkling that menopause would arrive so early for them. Pregnancy may still be possible, although it requires quick action and usually some help from medical science (see Chapter 6, "Fertility, Midlife, and Menopause Babies").

# Why Does Early Menopause Happen?

Sometimes it's easy to pinpoint the cause of early menopause, such as surgery that removes your ovaries. In such situations, you know that early menopause is imminent and you can prepare yourself. Other health factors, such as diabetes or treatment for cancer, can contribute to early menopause as well. For some women, family history plays a role as well. Sometimes the reason for early menopause is less definitive and may even remain a mystery.

## Surgery

With surgery that removes your ovaries (oopherectomy with or without hysterectomy) menopause is both inevitable and immediate. No ovaries, no eggs, and essentially no estrogen. It's the end of fertility, just like that. Surgery-induced early menopause can be more intense than normal menopause, not just because it's ahead of schedule, but because it happens without any of the typical preliminary changes that most women experience as perimenopause. Your body instead plunges into menopause, which can be quite a jolt.

Abdominal surgery that has nothing to do with your ovaries nonetheless can interrupt the blood flow to your ovaries, causing the sensitive follicles to wither and die.

It doesn't take much of an interruption to generate damage—it can even be microscopic. Because menopause occurs when your ovaries no longer produce eggs, fewer follicles mean that you'll reach this point earlier. Many doctors believe that this explains why early menopause seems to be more common among women who undergo a tubal ligation or a hysterectomy.

## Premature Ovarian Failure

Sometimes the ovaries just stop functioning for no apparent reason. When this happens in a woman under age 40, it's called *premature ovarian failure*. Although premature ovarian failure often results in premature or early menopause, the two are not necessarily the same. Premature ovarian failure can occur even before a woman starts menstruating, in which case it's usually called *primary amenorrhea*. In some women, premature ovarian failure comes and goes. These women may ovulate for several months and then not produce estrogen or have periods for up to a year. In the majority of women, however, the failure is permanent and menopause occurs.

Premature ovarian failure tends to surface when a woman is in her late 20s or early 30s, and it affects about 3 percent of American women. Many women discover the condition's existence when they stop taking birth control pills—and suddenly stop having periods. Women with premature ovarian failure may have fewer follicles than normal as a result of health problems or heredity. Or, their bodies may produce *antibodies* that attack their follicles and damage the eggs within them. About a third of women with this condition also have an *autoimmune disorder*.

Women with premature ovarian failure may have seemingly normal periods, too, which can add to the confusion. This is because their bodies continue to produce sufficient levels of progesterone to cause the lining of the uterus to build up each month. But their follicles aren't producing or

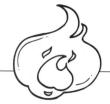

**Hot Flash!**

Doctors often recommend hormone replacement therapy for women who enter menopause in their 30s or 40s, to extend the protective qualities of estrogen. This helps hold at bay potentially serious medical problems such as osteoporosis and heart disease. If you are experiencing early menopause, be sure to discuss this with your doctor.

**Wise Up**

**Premature ovarian failure** exists when the ovaries stop functioning well ahead of the normal time of menopause, without precipitating medical conditions or surgery. **Primary amenorrhea** occurs when a young woman's menstrual periods never start, without the presence of any medical conditions that could cause amenorrhea (absence of menstruation).

### Wise Up

An **autoimmune disorder** is a health condition in which your body produces substances that attack its own tissues or organs. These substances are proteins called **antibodies**.

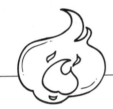

### Hot Flash!

Have you had your thyroid checked? Many of the signs of menopause—such as irregular periods, fatigue, depression, and weight gain—are also signs of hypothyroidism, or underactive thyroid. Many experts recommend that women who have these signs undergo blood tests to check their thyroid function, even if menopause appears to be obvious. Nearly 20 percent of women ages 60 and older have hypothyroidism.

releasing any eggs, so their cycles are empty, or anovulatory. As menopause approaches, they exhibit the usual signs of irregular periods because their hormone levels are fluctuating. It's just that these signs are a decade or two ahead of schedule.

Unless a woman is attempting to become pregnant, there's no medical reason to determine whether premature ovarian failure is the cause of early menopause. Any treatments for signs of menopause, such as hot flashes, are the same as they would be for menopause that was on schedule. Often, your doctor will check your follicle-stimulating hormone (FSH) levels to determine whether it is indeed early menopause. Diagnostic medical tests such as ovarian ultrasound or biopsy are not usually very helpful because their findings make no difference in terms of prospective treatment for either menopause signs or for infertility. Testing to determine a cause for early menopause is more useful for detecting other underlying medical conditions such as thyroid disorders.

Premature ovarian failure tends to strike women at an earlier age than other causes for early menopause, on average around age 27. This is often before women have had much opportunity to consider or plan becoming pregnant. Hormone replacement therapy can help some women with premature ovarian failure—usually those whose periods have stopped—establish ovulation for long enough to become pregnant. Conventional infertility treatments using other hormone drugs generally don't succeed.

## Autoimmune Disorders

A number of medical conditions involve your body turning on a part of itself. If you have one or more of these disorders, you might also find yourself dealing with early menopause. The most common autoimmune disorders are hypothyroidism (underactive or nonfunctioning thyroid gland), insulin-dependent diabetes (nonfunctioning pancreas), rheumatoid arthritis (inflammation and swelling of the joints), and systemic lupus erythematosus (inflammation of the connective tissues). Researchers don't fully understand how such conditions, called autoimmune disorders, develop. Many autoimmune disorders are significantly more common in women than in men, although doctors aren't sure why this is.

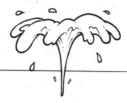

**Wellspring**

Women with insulin-dependent diabetes, also called type 1 diabetes (and formerly called juvenile or childhood-onset diabetes), are likely to experience menopause as much as 10 years early. This is partly the result of autoimmune activity and partly the result of the relationship between hormones and insulin. This relationship means that menopause also affects diabetes. When you have diabetes, your cells are less sensitive to the effects of insulin. But as progesterone levels fall off with the approach of menopause, insulin sensitivity increases. It can become difficult to maintain consistent blood sugar and blood insulin levels, requiring frequent insulin dose adjustments. Lifestyle factors such as exercise and diet are especially important during this transition. Once progesterone settles into its postmenopausal level, insulin levels again stabilize.

In some situations, such as hypothyroidism, treating the autoimmune disorder restores fertility in a woman who is chronologically young for menopause. In most cases, however, early menopause is permanent. Doctors believe that autoimmune activity accounts for about a third of all premature ovarian failure, which is a leading cause of early menopause.

## Polycystic Ovary Syndrome (PCOS)

Polycystic ovary syndrome (PCOS) is a metabolic condition in which the ovaries develop numerous cysts that interfere with follicle function and egg production. The ovaries produce more testosterone than they should, leading to irregular menstrual cycles as well as other symptoms such as male patterns of body hair and acne. The cysts often prevent the follicles from releasing eggs, so even when the woman has a period, she doesn't ovulate. PCOS is a leading cause of infertility in women and often sets the stage for early menopause when the scarred and damaged follicles stop functioning altogether.

Because irregular periods have marked their fertile years, women with PCOS might be uncertain about whether menopause is approaching. Other signs, such as hot flashes, night sweats, and mood swings, help mark the path more clearly. Consistently high FSH levels provide more tangible evidence. For some women with PCOS, early menopause is particularly traumatic because it closes the door on pregnancy. For others, menopause is a welcome transition because the PCOS goes away now that the hormone imbalances responsible for its symptoms no longer exist.

# A Family Affair

How old were your mother, grandmother, and any sisters who've preceded you in this life transition when they reached menopause? Many women tend to go through menopause at the same age their mothers did. This correlation seems stronger for women who experience menopause within the normal age range. Only about 5 percent of women who reach menopause early or prematurely have a family history of this pattern.

It's also possible for early menopause to be in your genes, which isn't quite the same thing as in your family history. Women who have defects involving an X chromosome, such as fragile X syndrome or Turner's syndrome, are more likely to have an early menopause. These defects tend to affect ovary development and ovulation as well.

# Cancer Treatment

Radiation therapy and chemotherapy to treat cancer often have the consequence of early menopause. When treatment is short-term, the effect can be temporary, with ovarian function stopping for a few months and then returning to normal. With full-course treatment, however, the stop is usually permanent. Doctors strive for a balance with chemotherapy and radiation therapy to find doses that kill cancer cells without killing too many healthy cells in the process. But although these therapies are improving in their ability to more narrowly target specific attributes of cancer cells, they still affect other cells. Ovarian cells are especially sensitive, making them vulnerable to damage.

Women who are at extraordinarily high risk for breast cancer may choose to take the chemotherapy agent *tamoxifen* in an effort to prevent breast cancer from developing. While this cuts their risk nearly in half, it significantly raises the probability of early menopause. Tamoxifen steps in to chemically take the place of estrogen, fooling the body into producing lower amounts of the real thing. Because estrogen fuels the growth of breast cancer cells, this cuts off the source. However, the masquerade has its limits. Tamoxifen may fool breast cancer cells, but it doesn't fool the ovaries. The reduced levels of estrogen signal the body to crank up FSH production. For many women, this initiates the sequence of changes leading to menopause. The transition is usually permanent and is not likely to reverse if the woman stops taking the tamoxifen.

**Wise Up**

**Tamoxifen** is a chemotherapy, or cancer treatment, drug that causes the body to produce less estrogen. It's often prescribed prophylactically (preventively) for women at high risk of breast cancer.

# Smoking: Guaranteed Early Menopause

Few things in life are certain. Taxes, car trouble when you're 2,000 miles from home, and rain on any day your plans are for outdoor activities rank right at the top of the list. If you smoke cigarettes, you can add a few more: starting your day with a 15-minute coughing spell, stopping to catch your breath after climbing any stairway with more than three steps, and ending your reproductive years well ahead of your nonsmoking peers.

Bluntly speaking, smoking is really good for nothing when it comes to your health. It has no known health benefits and leaves few, if any, body tissues and systems unharmed. The nicotine and other chemicals that you inhale with every drag from a cigarette clog your lungs, reducing their ability to get oxygen into your bloodstream. At the same time, these toxins cause your blood vessels—arteries, veins, and capillaries—to stiffen, which lessens their ability to transport blood to body tissues and cells. Your ovarian follicles are quite sensitive. When fluctuations in blood supply interrupt the flow of vital nutrients and oxygen to them, they die and your body cannot replace them. As a result, you run out of eggs ahead of schedule.

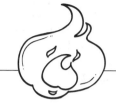

**Hot Flash!**

Some studies show that women who take HRT and smoke after menopause have lower levels of estrogen than women who take HRT and do not smoke. This further increases the risk of heart disease because smoking is itself a risk factor for heart disease.

For nearly all women who smoke, menopause comes at least two or three years early. For many, however, it arrives significantly sooner. It's not clear whether this is a lone consequence of smoking or the product of combined damage to the body, because smoking affects all body tissues. Cigarette smoking appears to lower a woman's estrogen levels, which may be another factor contributing to early menopause. Smoking affects the menopause experience of women smokers who enter menopause at a typical age, too, adding physical stresses that can worsen the normal signs of menopause and interfere with efforts to mitigate them.

# Stress-Induced Temporary Menopause

Doctors have long known that stress and your emotional state can affect your menstrual cycles, as you probably already know. Nearly every woman has at least one story of a late period she'll never forget, one fraught with worry and uncertainty about being pregnant. Some women have similar experiences when it comes to menopause. They may so dread or anticipate the approaching change in their lives that their emotions interfere with their physiology. Their periods may stop for several months, and they might have hot flashes and night sweats. Then just as suddenly as it all started, everything returns to normal.

Major physical or emotional trauma, such as serious injury or illness or the loss of a loved one, can also throw your body out of kilter, affecting not just your reproductive system, but other body systems as well. Most stress-induced menopause really isn't menopause at all, but rather an interruption of your body's nonvital functions while your body copes with whatever challenge is confronting it. Generally, when the stressor goes away, your periods return. Sometimes emotional trauma doesn't just go away. If your stress continues, a psychotherapist can often help you come to grips with your feelings.

# Navigating an Early Passage

For most women who experience it, early menopause is at the least a surprise. For some, especially those still planning to become pregnant, early menopause is an emotional shock. As with any transition, knowledge is power. The more you learn about menopause, the better able you are to navigate its passage. You wouldn't set out on a cross-country trip without some sense of where you were going and what possible challenges lay ahead! While you can't map your journey through menopause in the same way that you can plot your way along the highways, you can learn what to expect so that you're prepared for the changes your body encounters.

## *Coping with the Emotions*

Most women experience widely ranging emotions brought on by fluctuating hormone levels as they approach menopause, whether menopause occurs in midlife or arrives early. A woman's feelings about the transition of menopause add to the mix and can create a potent (and sometimes overwhelming) emotional environment. It helps tremendously to have a network of support—family and friends whom you trust and who care about you. These are the people who still love you when you complain and who reassure you that this, too, shall pass, and your life will eventually return to normal.

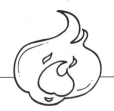

**Hot Flash!**

Depression is more than the blues that affect everyone at some time. If you find yourself with little interest in eating or getting out of bed in the morning, and unable to enjoy the things in your life that once brought you pleasure, see your doctor. Depression is a treatable medical condition.

What do you do when your family and friends think you're overly emotional about your early menopause passage, or you find you are having trouble communicating your thoughts and feelings to someone who will not only listen but *understand?* Misunderstandings and miscommunications are unfortunate, but they sometimes happen when the people around you have different perceptions of how your menopause experience should be, or are dismissive of your thoughts and feelings about it. You can do yourself a great deal of good by seeking knowledgeable support, perhaps through a support group, conversations with your doctor, or sessions with a licensed counselor or psychotherapist. It's important to express your emotions—be tenacious in making a connection to someone who can help you work through this passage.

## Facing the End of Your Childbearing Years

The loss of childbearing potential can be a traumatic event no matter how old you are when you reach menopause. For women who experience this transition while friends and relatives their age are having babies, the unexpected and premature end of fertility can be emotionally devastating. It's normal to feel a strong and even severe sense of loss, just as you might feel pain at the loss of a loved one. If you haven't yet completed or even started your family, early menopause means that you're not likely to have biological children. It's normal to experience grief over this loss, and it's important to allow yourself to acknowledge and experience your grief.

Grief is a process that can take weeks, months, or years to work through. It's normal to pass through several stages, from denial and anger to eventual acceptance. Even when they're no longer grieving, many people still feel a sense of sadness. Many hospitals and health organizations sponsor support groups where people with similar circumstances can come together to share their feelings and experiences. This can help you cope with your emotions and grief.

How long your cycle of grief lasts is very personal. Some women complete the cycle quite quickly, arriving at acceptance before their bodies reach the completion of menopause. Even though menopause comes early for them, they reach a level of comfort about this new stage in their lives with relative ease. One end of the continuum is not necessarily better than the other. What is good, and what is normal, is what works for you.

Sometimes grief is a life-altering circumstance. Early menopause alters the normal life cycle, and as a result presents unique challenges that can continue to affect you long after menopause is complete. It's important for most women facing this situation to have others in their lives—partners, family, friends—understand and appreciate that this isn't just about menopause.

### Embracing Change

Early menopause might mean that you can no longer conceive biological children, but it doesn't mean that your parenting options are completely dissolved. Donor egg and adoption remain possibilities for those who still want to create families.

## Age: The Clash of Biology and Chronology

Early or premature menopause does not mean that you're aging faster! It just means that your ovaries left work early. The rest of your body stays on schedule. It's interesting that while life expectancy has nearly doubled over the last 100 years, the average

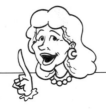

age of menopause has remained relatively the same. This is one of the many mysteries that researchers hope to someday unravel in the quest to understand aging.

Early menopause means only that your ovaries have stopped functioning ahead of schedule. Because estrogen seems to play a role in holding heart disease and osteoporosis at bay, it's important for you to take other steps to keep your risks for these potentially serious health problems as low as possible. Eat a low-fat diet, get plenty of regular exercise (aerobic and weight-bearing), don't smoke, and drink alcohol in moderation if you drink at all. With early menopause, you'll have more years without your body's natural estrogen. If you take good care of yourself, your body won't complain!

## Should You Attempt to Delay Early Menopause?

Because early menopause appears to be an unnatural event according to Mother Nature's timetable, it's a natural reaction to turn to medical technology for help in restoring this transition to its normal schedule. Unfortunately, however, doctors usually can do little to delay early menopause. As we mentioned earlier, HRT sometimes restores ovulation in women with premature ovarian failure, holding off menopause. Treating underlying medical conditions such as hypothyroidism also sometimes returns menstruation to its normal pattern.

Recently, doctors have started experimenting with ovarian grafts, surgically implanting healthy ovarian tissue onto damaged or diseased ovaries. Results are very preliminary and so far have involved removing and freezing a woman's ovarian tissue before a procedure such as chemotherapy or radiation therapy, and then surgically replanting the tissue following the treatment. Although there is great hope for its success in restoring fertility for women facing early menopause, researchers are less certain that ovarian grafting could indefinitely delay menopause regardless of a woman's age.

It's often difficult to accept that your body is preparing to end its fertile years at the same time the bodies of friends who are your age are preparing for pregnancy and birth. At some point in the future, perhaps it will be possible to reset your biological clock. Researchers continue to explore the reasons and the processes of early menopause.

### The Least You Need to Know

➤ Most often, there is no single, clearly identifiable cause for early menopause.

➤ About a third of women who reach menopause early have premature ovarian failure—their ovaries quit working.

➤ Most efforts to delay menopause are unsuccessful.

➤ Physically, early menopause is usually no more difficult a transition than menopause that arrives on schedule.

➤ Emotionally, early menopause can present significant challenges.

# Part 3

# Ch-Ch-Changes:
# Menopause Symptoms

*Change is not new to you, of course. Indeed, it's probably the one constant in your life. But there has never been a change quite like this one. When you emerge from the turbulence of the next five or six years, you'll feel like a new woman. As some experiences and life options draw to a close, others open up. Each woman's path is at once unique and universal. Your menopause experience will be a lot like, but still different from, your mother's or your best friend's or your neighbor's.*

*The chapters in this part take a look at the changes that you can expect and that you might encounter on your journey through menopause.*

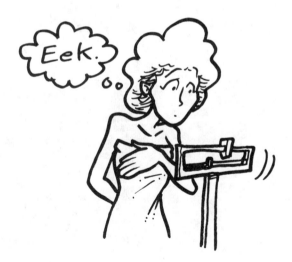

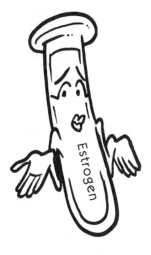

# Chapter 9

# Hormones for Healthy Menopause

---

**In This Chapter**

➤ Menopause as a condition

➤ Menopause as a transition

➤ Your hormone quotient: a self-quiz

➤ How stress affects the experience of menopause

➤ How hormone balance affects the signs of menopause

---

You might say that hormones usher in every major life change you experience. From conception to old age, these chemical messengers signal various body systems to accelerate, maintain, or diminish their functions. Puberty, the onset of sexual maturity, is a key hormonal threshold that both women and men remember. While men generally can forget about their hormones once past this rite of passage (at least for several decades), women face monthly reminders of theirs.

For better or for worse, hormones become the life partners that establish your sense of womanliness. You settle into the pattern of their companionship, knowing that changes in the pattern herald major changes in life.

# Condition or Transition: Taking a Point of View on Menopause

When scientists reported the first successful graft of a human ovary in 1999, a wave of wonder splashed around the world. Could this be the "cure" for menopause? A tsunami of questions and dialogue followed. Is menopause something that needs to be cured? Just because medical science can alter the course of nature, should it? Two camps of opinion emerged: those who felt that the hormonal shifts of menopause represented a medical problem in need of fixing, and those who felt that the hormonal shifts of menopause were a normal and natural dimension of growing older worthy of celebration.

# Condition: Menopause Is About Hormonal Imbalances

In our medicalized modern Western culture, many of the life events that hormones orchestrate have become conditions. Menstruation, pregnancy, and menopause all "require" medical monitoring, if not intervention. While menstruation and pregnancy reflect hormonal cycles, in this view, menopause indicates a hormonal imbalance in need of restoration. Just as doctors might prescribe hormone replacement for a pancreas or a thyroid gland that stops functioning, goes the argument, they also should prescribe hormone replacement when the ovaries shut down their production. After all, the correlation between estrogen and potentially life-threatening medical problems such as heart disease and osteoporosis establishes this hormone as every bit as essential as insulin (produced by the pancreas) and thyroxin (produced by the thyroid gland). Why shouldn't doctors treat this loss in the same way?

The key difference is that not every woman experiences loss of thyroid function (*hypothyroidism*) or pancreas function (*insulin-dependent diabetes*), but every woman who lives to midlife does experience a dramatic reduction in estrogen production that results in menopause. Diabetes, of course, is life-threatening without treatment. Untreated hypothyroidism leads to a myriad of other medical problems. Treatment eases great discomfort for many women, to be sure. But unlike the symptoms of diabetes and hypothyroidism, which worsen unless they are treated, the signs of menopause eventually end with or without treatment.

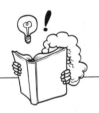

**Wise Up**

**Hypothyroidism** is a medical condition in which the thyroid gland fails to produce adequate levels of thyroxin and other hormones. **Insulin-dependent diabetes** is a medical condition in which the pancreas stops producing the hormone insulin.

Medical science has much to offer in the way of relief for the signs of menopause, of course. Ignoring this can be foolhardy and can subject a woman to unnecessary discomfort and suffering. Every woman needs to evaluate her unique and specific needs and circumstances, and make decisions based on what will work best for her. The issue is not whether medical intervention helps make the transition easier (it certainly can, and it does for thousands of women). Rather, the question is whether medical intervention is necessary for every woman. Although readjusting the body's hormones through supplements restores the hormonal balance, it doesn't restore the reproductive system's primary function: fertility. Once those eggs are gone, they're gone—no amount of hormonal supplementation is going to bring them back or make more. There are still many unanswered questions about the long-term effects of hormone replacement therapy—as well as about the long-term effects of estrogen depletion.

To some extent, many of us find it relieving to know we can count on our doctors to offer treatments for menopause and its discomforts. In a culture where it's possible to get nearly anything from a burger to a home loan in a matter of minutes, we've come to expect instant cures for whatever ails us. And doctors, being the kind of people who want to help others feel better, often feel obligated to give us what we request (or demand). It's a challenge to maintain a balance between competing needs.

## *Transition: Menopause Is About Hormonal Shifts*

Many cultures around the world celebrate the life events that hormones orchestrate, including menstruation and menopause. In such cultures, for example, Japan, the signs of menopause seem to be far less disruptive for women than in our Western culture. Some experts speculate that this is as much biological as it is cultural, pointing out that women in other parts of the world tend to eat a more vegetarian diet than is common in the United States. Particularly in Japan and other Eastern cultures, the diet is high in soy products that are rich in *phytoestrogens*. This provides a natural source of hormone supplementation, according to this view, suppressing many of menopause's uncomfortable signs such as hot flashes.

It's likely, however, that attitude plays just as important a role in how menopause affects a woman as do other factors such as hormone levels and lifestyle. We've known for a long time that knowledge is power—a person who understands as much as possible about what's going on with his or her body is less likely to feel anxious or out-of-control than someone who knows very little about body functions. The mind/body connection is a powerful and not fully understood dimension of health and healing. We know, for example, that stress is a factor in many health conditions, from headache to high blood pressure. We also know that activities that rely on the natural integration of the body, mind, and spirit (that are biopsychophysical)—such as meditation, yoga, and biofeedback—often can alter or relieve such conditions.

**Wise Up**

**Phytoestrogens** are substances chemically similar to estrogen that come from certain plants and seeds. Soybeans are a natural source of phytoestrogens, as are sunflower seeds and bean sprouts.

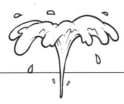

### Wellspring

A number of studies have demonstrated that surgery patients handle pain much better when they know how much pain to expect and how long it will last. The fear of pain is often worse than the pain itself. Surgeons and anesthesiologists now make it standard practice to discuss pain and pain relief with patients before surgery. Many recovery rooms use patient-controlled analgesia (PCA) to let patients administer their own intravenous pain medication as they need it. Studies show that patients report a higher level of relief and comfort, and use less pain medication when they control when and how much medication they receive.

# What's Your Hormone Quotient? A Self-Quiz

In a recent study reported by the American Society for Reproductive Medicine, nearly two thirds of the women surveyed did not know what hormones played roles in menopause. How well do you know your hormones? Choose the correct answer for each of the following questions.

1. A woman's main sex hormones are …
   a. Estrogen, progesterone, and testosterone
   b. Estrogen, hydrocortisone, and aldosterone
   c. ACTH, TSH, and FSH
   d. Progesterone, prolactin, and oxytocin

2. As menopause approaches, a woman's body …
   a. Increases progesterone and estrogen production
   b. Increases progesterone and decreases estrogen production
   c. Decreases progesterone and increases estrogen production
   d. Decreases progesterone and estrogen production

3. The hormone responsible for hot flashes is …
   a. Progesterone
   b. Testosterone
   c. Estrogen
   d. Epinephrine

4. Hot flashes occur because the amount of the hormone responsible for them ...

    a. Increases

    b. Decreases

    c. Fluctuates

    d. Stays the same while other hormone levels decrease

5. Your ovaries produce these hormones:

    a. Just progesterone

    b. Just estrogen

    c. Estrogen and progesterone

    d. Estrogen, progesterone, and testosterone

6. The hormone primarily responsible for a woman's sex drive is ...

    a. Estrogen

    b. Progesterone

    c. Testosterone

    d. Epinephrine

7. When estrogen levels fall, a woman's body increases its production of ...

    a. Insulin

    b. Progesterone

    c. Estrogen

    d. FSH

8. When a woman is pregnant, the organ that produces the hormones that sustain the pregnancy is ...

    a. Pancreas

    b. Parathyroid gland

    c. Placenta

    d. Adrenal gland

9. The hormone that causes the lining of the uterus to thicken and then slough during the menstrual cycle is ...

    a. Estrogen

    b. Progesterone

    c. Testosterone

    d. FSH

10. The hormone that seems to offer a woman protection against heart disease and osteoporosis is ...

    a. FSH

    b. Progesterone

    c. Estrogen

    d. Hydrocortisone

11. Women with high percentages of body fat are more likely than women with low percentages of body fat to have higher levels of this hormone following menopause:

    a. Progesterone

    b. Testosterone

    c. Estrogen

    d. Epinephrine

12. Recent research suggests that there might be a link between this hormone and Alzheimer's disease in women who are past menopause:

    a. Estrogen

    b. Progesterone

    c. Testosterone

    d. FSH

Ready to see how much you know about your hormones? Here are the answers:

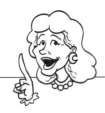

**Wise Woman's Wisdom**

"There is a fountain of youth: It is your mind, your talents, the creativity you bring to your life and the lives of the people you love. When you learn to tap this source, you will truly have defeated age."

—Sophia Loren

1. **The correct answer is a.** A woman's main sex hormones are estrogen, progesterone, and, yes, testosterone, which we traditionally think of as a male hormone.

2. **The correct answer is b.** As menopause approaches, a woman's body decreases production of both progesterone and estrogen.

3. **The correct answer is c.** Estrogen is responsible for the hot flashes many women experience as they approach menopause.

4. **The correct answer is c.** Hot flashes occur when estrogen levels fluctuate.

5. **The correct answer is d.** Your ovaries produce estrogen, progesterone, and testosterone, a woman's three main sex hormones.

6. **The correct answer is c.** Although it's only present in tiny amounts, testosterone is the hormone responsible for a woman's sex drive.

7. **The correct answer is d.** When estrogen levels fall, a woman's body increases its production of FSH in an effort to cause the ovary's follicle to release an egg to begin the menstrual cycle again.

8. **The correct answer is c.** When a woman is pregnant, the placenta is largely responsible for producing the hormones that sustain the pregnancy. Numerous hormonal changes throughout the body also contribute.

9. **The correct answer is b.** The hormone that causes the lining of the uterus to thicken and then slough during the menstrual cycle is progesterone.

10. **The correct answer is c.** The hormone that seems to offer a woman protection against heart disease and osteoporosis is estrogen. However, emerging evidence indicates that while testosterone increases the risk of heart disease, it decreases the risk of osteoporosis.

11. **The correct answer is c.** Women with high percentages of body fat are more likely than women with low percentages of body fat to have higher levels of estrogen following menopause. This is because fat cells store and produce small amounts of estrogen.

12. **The correct answer is a.** Recent research suggests that there might be a link between estrogen and Alzheimer's disease in women who are past menopause. Estrogen has many and varied roles in a woman's health.

Do you know as much as you thought you knew? If you got eight or more answers correct, you know more about hormones than the average woman. If you got six or more answers correct, you're off to a good start, although you could use some extra study time. And if you got five or fewer answers correct, bone up by reading the next section!

# Endocrinology 101: A Quick Review

While discussions about menopause and hormones tend to focus on the ovaries, the functions of other endocrine glands play a role as well. The adrenal glands, a pair of spongelike clusters of tissue, drape over the top of each kidney. The outer portion of the adrenal gland, called the adrenal cortex, secrete a number of important hormones, including

**Embracing Change**

Regular exercise is one of the best ways to help your body function as efficiently as possible. Just walking for 30 minutes at a time, three or four days a week, helps keep your metabolism up. Exercise is also a wonderful stress reliever, letting you work off the steam that has built up from the day's pressures.

hydrocortisone (cortisol), aldosterone, and androgens (testosterone and DHEA). The inner core of the adrenal gland, called the adrenal medulla, secretes epinephrine and norepinephrine. The adrenal glands take their marching orders from a part of the brain called the hypothalamus and from another endocrine gland, the pituitary gland.

These structures work in concert to maintain the right balance of hormones for your body's state of affairs. Because your body's status shifts literally by the minute depending on the time of day and what you're doing, this system stays quite busy. Epinephrine and cortisol are key players in your body's stress response, while the androgens affect (and are affected by) ovarian function.

## Stress and Menopause

Stress produces a physiological reaction that puts your body on alert. In the short term, this is not always a bad thing—stress is a normal and useful response to situations demanding your immediate attention. In a carryover of the primal fight-or-flight reaction, stress prepares your body systems to either fight or flee for your safety or life in threatening situations. In response to such a threat, real or perceived, your adrenal glands send a flood of hormones, with cortisol and epinephrine in the lead, into your body to prime key systems for peak performance. Your heart rate, blood pressure, and breathing rate all jump. Your metabolism steps up the pace, bringing more oxygen and other nutrients to muscle and nerve cells that might need to get you moving in a hurry.

Now if you're fending off the advances of an attacking saber tooth tiger, this response is a good thing—and very likely your only chance to see another sunrise. But the challenges of our modern world are considerably more sedentary than were the conflicts that confronted our ancestors. You're more apt to be dodging verbal bullets in a meeting or stuck in bumper-to-bumper traffic crawling toward your destination at the pace of a speeding snail than fighting for your life.

The sometimes drastic drops in estrogen that often occur as your body prepares for menopause can trigger the same fight-or-flight response from your body as the charge of a hungry tiger might. This reflects the intricate and delicate balance among your body's hormones. The actions of one trigger a sequence of actions in the others.

## Healthy Amounts of Cortisol and DHEA

DHEA is a naturally occurring hormone that the body converts into estrogen and testosterone. It reaches its peak level when you're in your mid-20s and steadily declines after then. While doctors don't entirely understand the role of DHEA, they do know that people with osteoporosis have lower than normal levels of this hormone. Cortisol is the body's natural form of hydrocortisone. Your adrenal glands release cortisol in response to stress to fortify your immune system. When cortisol levels remain high, your stress response stays high. Instead of strengthening your immune system as intended, a perpetually high cortisol level instead may weaken it. High cortisol levels are linked to a number of health problems, including heart disease and cancer.

The relationship between cortisol and DHEA is one that researchers are studying with great interest. A rise in cortisol levels and a drop in DHEA levels seems to herald a change in health condition. Maintaining a balance between these two hormones could be the key to preventing a number of diseases, although much study remains to be done. The jury is still out on the safety and value of taking DHEA supplements. Because these products are classified as nutritional supplements rather than drugs, they are not subject to the federal standards for testing that drugs must pass before being approved for sale in the United States. The amount of DHEA that's beneficial seems to be highly individual, and too much DHEA can translate into problems associated with high levels of androgen such as male body hair patterns (hirsuitism). We discuss DHEA, cortisol, and other substances taken as supplements to relieve the signs of menopause in Part 4, "HRT or No HRT, That Is the Question."

## *Estrogen, Progesterone, and FSH*

These three hormones form the core of menopause. As you might remember from Chapter 5, "Menopause and Your Body," your ovaries produce varying levels of estrogen and progesterone at different stages of your menstrual cycle. These three hormones work closely with each other, orchestrating the events of ovulation and menstruation. As the number of viable follicles diminishes, estrogen production and then progesterone production fall off while FSH production skyrockets. The smooth cycle of fertility becomes an endless loop. Eventually your body stabilizes with high FSH levels and low levels of estrogen and progesterone.

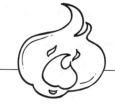

**Hot Flash!**

Talk with your doctor before you start taking nutritional supplements containing DHEA. Each person needs and uses DHEA at an individual level. A quantity of DHEA that's too high for you can cause more problems than it solves.

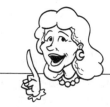

**Wise Woman's Wisdom**

"You don't get to choose how you're going to die, or when. You can only decide how you're going to live now."

—Joan Baez

# Are Balanced Hormones the Solution to Menopause?

Doctors don't entirely understand the relationship between the hormone changes that result in menopause and the signs of menopause. Estrogen takes the heat for triggering many of the short-term experiences such as hot flashes and mood swings. However, some studies suggest that DHEA and cortisol play an equally important role and may also contribute to long-term problems such as memory loss, osteoporosis, and heart disease. None of these signs and symptoms exist in most younger women when their fertility hormones are in balance. This causes doctors to question whether restoring this balance—in ratios, if not in levels—could indefinitely suspend menopause.

Part of the answer lies in how we interpret the role and meaning of menopause. Unlike osteoporosis or heart disease, menopause itself is not a sign of damage to the body. Even though the risk for these health problems dramatically increases after menopause, doctors aren't entirely sure whether the increase is related to the hormonal changes of menopause or is simply a function of aging. After all, hormones rage during adolescence, too, yet there are few arguments for "fixing" that transition (pleas from the parents of adolescents notwithstanding).

## How Hormonal Balance Can Relieve Menopause Signs

Many women experience great relief from signs such as hot flashes, night sweats, and mood swings when they begin hormone replacement therapy (HRT). Once their estrogen levels begin to rise, the hormonal cycles wreaking havoc with their bodies abate. This relief generally carries through the period of time, usually three to six years, that your body is preparing for menopause. Once menopause has occurred—you've had your last period—hormonal balance naturally shifts and signs such as hot flashes go away.

## How Hormonal Balance Can Exacerbate Menopause Signs

Attempting to restore the body's balance of hormones can have the unintended result of worsening, rather than improving, the signs of menopause. Synthetic progesterone supplements, typically a part of HRT for a woman who still has her uterus, can cause regular or irregular bleeding that rivals menstruation. It can also produce world-class PMS symptoms that are far worse for some women than those they experienced while they were menstruating.

Some women worry about selectively replacing hormones. Doctors are only just beginning to unravel the intricate interactions among the body's natural hormones, and they don't yet fully understand the very long-term ramifications of replacing the body's natural hormones with synthetic substitutes. Typical HRT replaces just estrogen and progesterone but does not restore fertility (with the exception of some women with premature ovarian failure, in whom HRT can stimulate ovulation because their ovaries still have some eggs). Although this suppresses the unpleasant signs of menopause, it doesn't alter the reality of physiology that's behind menopause: Your body has run out of eggs.

# Finding *Your* Balance Between Condition and Transition

Although menopause is an experience common to all women who reach midlife, it is nonetheless an individual and unique adventure for each woman. For some women, the signs of menopause are so severe that they interfere with other life activities. Other women barely notice them. If there is a single message about menopause that meets with no argument, it's that each woman needs to assess her own situation and make decisions about her transition through menopause based on her experiences and feelings. While no one approach fits every woman, each woman can find an approach that fits her.

## The Least You Need to Know

➤ Normal menopause, like adolescence, is more about transitions than medical conditions.

➤ Stress can dramatically shift the experience and signs of menopause.

➤ Numerous hormones beyond the traditional "female" hormones play a role in menopause.

➤ Menopause is at once an experience common to all women and an adventure unique to each woman.

# Chapter 10

# A Shift from Left Brain to Right Brain

---

### In This Chapter

➤ How your left brain works

➤ How your right brain works

➤ Which part of your brain leads you? A self-quiz

➤ How to develop your nondominant brain

➤ Developing and using your intuition

---

A funny thing happens on your way to menopause. You have days when you forget where you're going or what you intend to do when you arrive. A friend you've known since Girl Scouts suddenly becomes a stranger when it's time to introduce her to someone else. The numbers in your checkbook turn into hieroglyphics, forming an amusing pattern or picture that causes you to laugh out loud right there in the supermarket checkout line. The tempest of your shifting hormones rearranges your thought patterns and processes much as a tornado rearranges the landscape, leaving you feeling confused and betrayed. Don't worry—this is all perfectly normal. You're not losing your mind. In fact, it's more likely that you're finding parts of your mind that you didn't know you had.

Your brain is a mysterious and amazing blend of physiology and chemistry. It handles the functions of both intellect (thinking) and emotion (feeling). Specialized nerve cells called neurons serve as the highways and side streets along which chemical messengers zoom as they travel between parts of your brain and parts of your body. In some respects, menopause hits your brain like rush hour hits Los Angeles. Everything moves along just fine, and then all of a sudden there's more traffic than the network can handle. Conduits clog, and messages get jammed up or misdirected. When this happens on the interstate, you could end up late for a meeting or appointment. When it happens in your brain, you could have trouble remembering or thinking clearly.

# How Your Brain Thinks

Busy organ that it is, your brain's *cerebrum* dedicates certain areas of itself to specific functions. The separation of responsibilities starts with a literal partition in the brain's physical structure. Split lengthwise down the center, the brain divides into the right and left hemispheres. The nerve signals from each cross at the top of the spinal cord before going out to the body. This means that the right hemisphere controls the functions of the left side of the body, while the left controls the functions of the right side of the body. This cross-control remains an invisible aspect of human physiology until something goes wrong, such as a stroke. Damage to the right hemisphere shows up as disability on the left side of the body, and vice versa.

**Wise Up**

The **cerebrum** is the largest and most developed of the three physical parts of the human brain. A conglomerate of nerve cells and fibers, the cerebrum handles all conscious and mental processes, including thought and memory.

Beyond their physical separation from one another, each half of the brain has a mind of its own, so to speak. The left brain excels in linear thought. It processes language and words, analyzes arithmetic equations, applies logic to problem solving, and organizes. It thrives on planning and order. The right brain shines in creativity. It perceives the tones and inflections of language, expresses imagination, and envisions the world in three-dimensional images. It flourishes on randomness and chaos.

While the two sides of your brain—the right brain and the left brain—combine forces to present a more or less whole perspective of the world around you, one side is usually dominant. You hear and understand speech, for example, although you may respond more to intonations (right brain) or to grammatical structure (left brain). In an argument, you might find logic (left brain) more persuasive than emotion (right brain). We all need both right and left brain functions to properly interpret the world around us. Your brain is a prime example of how the whole is greater than the sum of its parts.

## *Your Analytical Left Brain*

When it's time to balance your checkbook, plan a family reunion, or organize the supply closet, your left brain rolls into action. Many everyday activities rely on the left brain for its skills in organizing, planning, analyzing, and calculating. For much of our lives, we're encouraged to use and develop these skills that our culture values. The left brain likes order and sequence, the key attributes of logic and linear thinking. It gets you to work on time, properly dressed and equipped with all that you need to start your day. People who are dominantly left-brained often find happiness in careers such as accounting and bookkeeping, engineering, and technology. Many become doctors, lawyers, pharmacists, managers, or administrators.

## Your Creative Right Brain

Sprawled comfortably on the other side of your brain is your carefree creativity. This primary function of the right brain is continually at work gathering information and collecting input. (You wouldn't know this from looking at a right-brained person, who often appears to be daydreaming or lost in another world.) While your left brain looks at the clouds and analyzes the probability that they'll dump rain on the afternoon's plans, your right brain gazes into the sky and sees knights jousting or a lion chasing an elephant. Conceptual activities such as music and writing draw from the right brain's abilities. Your right brain knows few boundaries. It generates original and daring ideas. People who are dominantly right-brained often explore careers that feature variety, creativity, and unpredictability. They are often entrepreneurs, artists, nurses, or psychiatrists.

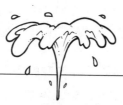

### Wellspring

No one is entirely certain why about 1 in 10 people is left-handed, although research indicates that it could be because they're right-brained. Several theories link handedness to the location of the speech center (also called Broca's area) in the brain. In most people who are right-handed, the speech center resides in the left side of the brain. In most left-handed people, the speech center resides in the right side of the brain. A number of the world's most creative people have been left-handed—among them Michelangelo, Leonardo da Vinci, Pablo Picasso, Isaac Newton, and Albert Einstein. Some researchers believe this suggests that the more completely one side of the brain dominates, the more intense the characteristics of that domination are.

# Are Women Right More Often Than Men?

Some experts believe that gender influences brain dominance. Men, they say, tend to approach the world in linear fashion. In her book *The First Sex* (Random House, 1999), anthropologist Helen Fisher describes her observation that men's brains think in a linear progression of steps, while women's brains think in what she describes as "webs of interrelated factors." Men focus on the parts, Fisher says, while women focus on the whole or how the parts relate to the whole. Although Fisher views these distinctions in the context of human development, they also epitomize left brain/right brain dominance. Of course, such characterizations are generalities. There are right-brained men just as there are left-brained women. Cultural and social roles make it difficult to determine whether apparent gender differences in thinking patterns arise from nature or necessity.

Research into how brain functions change with aging suggests that necessity has the edge. In one study that compared typing ability between college students and people over age 60 (all excellent typists), the oldsters had little trouble keeping up with the youngsters. While the college students had greater physical agility and faster reaction times (left brain), both men and women in the group of elders exchanged deficiencies in these areas for efficiencies in their actions and approach (right brain). In other words, the older group was more creative in problem solving, looking beyond the obvious "right" answer to find other solutions. From an anthropology perspective, this ability to adapt improves survivability. It could be that the apparent mind-shifts of menopause are part of the inherent human design to lengthen longevity and improve the odds in competition with others who are younger.

# Left or Right, What's Your Style? A Self-Quiz

Is your perspective left or right? This self-quiz can give you some insight into how your brain processes information. For each question or statement, select the response that most closely describes you. There are no right or wrong answers (just right and left!).

1. When I meet someone new, I form an opinion about him or her …
   a. After we've been together several times and I know more about him or her
   b. Instantly, based on my gut instincts
   c. It depends on the person and the situation
2. When I look at those pictures that are patterns of dots, I see …
   a. Patterns of dots
   b. Three-dimensional images
   c. Dots and patterns shifting back and forth
3. When I have to solve a challenging problem, I …
   a. Sit at my desk and outline everything I know about the situation, then move through my outline step by step

      **b.** Go for a walk, take a shower, or do something else that has no particular purpose

      **c.** It depends on the problem

4. Rules …

      **a.** Should always be followed

      **b.** Are made to be broken

      **c.** Establish order and structure

5. When assembling toys, models, or furniture from a kit, I …

      **a.** Lay out all the parts in the order the instructions tell me I'll use them, and then follow the directions to assemble the item

      **b.** Empty out all the parts and then start putting the item together

      **c.** Read through the instructions and then start assembling the item; if I run into trouble, I'll look at the instructions again

6. If someone walked into my office or home right now, he or she would find …

      **a.** A place for everything and everything in its place

      **b.** Nothing unless he or she knew exactly where to look

      **c.** Reasonable order and tidiness, with a few papers or magazines lying around

7. I prefer instructions that …

      **a.** Are written

      **b.** Show pictures

      **c.** Combine words and pictures

8. When cooking according to a recipe, I …

      **a.** Prepare and organize all the ingredients on the counter according to the order I'll use them, and measure everything

      **b.** Guesstimate the amounts because I've lost my measuring spoons, and run to the store to pick up any ingredients I'm missing

      **c.** Substitute ingredients depending on what's in my cupboard or what taste variations appeal to me

9. On rainy days, I like to …

      **a.** Clean closets

      **b.** Sit at the window to watch and listen to the rain

      **c.** Read or do some sort of craft

10. When a recipe or a project doesn't turn out as intended, I …

      **a.** Retrace my steps to figure out where I went wrong

      **b.** Laugh at the absurd results

      **c.** See what I can do to fix or make other use of the results

11. When I drive on vacation, I ...

    **a.** Mark my route on the map, plan how far I'll drive each day, and make motel reservations in advance

    **b.** Stop in little towns and tourist attractions along the way, detour if the road looks more interesting than the one I'm on, and stop for the night when I'm tired

    **c.** Look at the map before I leave, and write myself a few notes about key turns and distances

12. When the telephone rings, I ...

    **a.** Always answer it

    **b.** Let it ring if I'm busy or don't feel like talking

    **c.** Screen calls through my answering machine

Do you think of yourself as right-brained, left-brained, or pretty balanced? If you have seven or more As, your left brain takes control of most aspects of your life. If you have seven or more Bs, your right brain runs the show. If you have an equal number of As and Bs, or seven or more Cs, your right- and left-brain functions balance for a whole-brain approach to thinking (more on this a little later in this chapter).

## Estrogen and Short-Term Memory

You can't find your car keys. You drive to the store and then can't remember what you need to buy. Your mind goes blank when someone asks for your address or phone number. What's happening to your memory? It could well be reacting to the drop in estrogen levels that your body experiences with menopause. Some researchers believe that estrogen functions as a facilitator, directing the traffic of memory information to and from your brain's memory centers. When estrogen levels fall below a certain point, the transfer process becomes sluggish and disorganized. The result: You know you remember something, but you can't quite remember what it is.

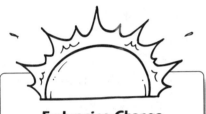

**Embracing Change**

Just as physical exercise keeps your body in shape, mental exercise can keep your mind in top form. Doing crossword puzzles, playing card and board games, reading, and playing a musical instrument are among the many mental activities that give your brain a good workout.

## Memory Challenges During Menopause

Many women experience changes in short-term memory during menopause. Experts disagree about whether this is primarily the result of dropping estrogen levels or other factors. Menopause is often a time of high stress in a woman's life, as many life changes beyond hormones are taking place. Children are often leaving home, and women may find themselves questioning career and relationship choices. These changes are stressful, and stress affects many functions, including cognition (the ability to think) and memory. Tipping the scales of evidence more toward estrogen's role, however, is evidence that memory and thinking ability often improve when a woman takes HRT. For most women, the challenges that surface as a result of menopause are temporary—with or without HRT. The story could be different for challenges that occur later in life, long after menopause.

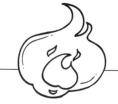

**Hot Flash!**

Changes in estrogen levels are by no means the only reason or explanation for memory and thinking problems. If you continue to have trouble with these functions, see your doctor to rule out other causes.

## Estrogen, Memory Loss, and Alzheimer's Disease

Some evidence suggests that estrogen replacement therapy can slow the progress of Alzheimer's disease. This has led to hope that estrogen might also delay or prevent this progressive, debilitating disease that affects more than four million Americans. Alzheimer's disease is difficult to diagnose, with autopsy after death being the only certain measure of the disorder's presence. In a normal brain, chemicals called neurotransmitters conduct signals between neurons, or nerve cells. People who have Alzheimer's disease have extremely low levels of the neurotransmitter that plays a key role in memory, acetycholine.

## HRT and Memory Improvement

Women taking HRT noticed that as their hot flashes disappeared, their memories returned. Researchers began to explore the connection between estrogen and memory. Although researchers don't yet understand how or why, estrogen also appears to facilitate communication between neurons, sort of chemically greasing the rails to make travel faster and easier for neurotransmitters. It looks like estrogen might also increase the levels of acetycholine in the brain, as well as the levels of other key neurotransmitters such as dopamine (linked to mood and thought) and serotonin (linked to mood). A number of studies underway are seeking to further isolate and identify the function of estrogen in memory and Alzheimer's disease.

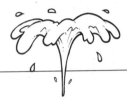

**Wellspring**

Many factors other than estrogen are involved with Alzheimer's disease, of course. The brains of people with Alzheimer's disease show characteristic damage. Deposits called neuritic plaques coat clusters of nerve cells. The plaques interfere with the cells' ability to communicate with one another by blocking the synapses, or spaces between them. The fibers within neurons, which in a healthy brain are straight and parallel to each other like microscopic railroad tracks, become tangled (called neurofibrillary tangles). Evidence also indicates that there are genetic factors involved. Alzheimer's disease, especially early on-set, seems to run in families. In addition, people with Down's syndrome, a genetic defect involving chromosome 21, have a high risk of developing Alzheimer's disease.

# Thinking Outside the Box: Nonlinear Thought

Most of us are programmed to look for *the* right answer to a problem. But in reality, most life situations have multiple right answers. The trick is to open yourself to the possibilities. Motivational speakers like to tell the tale of two frogs who, while hopping around the farm one day, jumped into a bucket of fresh cream. One frog tried again and again to climb up the bucket's steep, straight sides but kept sliding back into the bucket. Exhausted, the frog accepted its fate and sank to the bottom. The other frog kept swimming around in circles, kicking with long, vigorous strokes. Just as the frog was getting too tired to continue, it noticed large lumps beginning to form. Before long the second frog had churned the cream to butter, gained a foothold, and leaped out of the bucket. Although this was not the answer the frog expected, it was the solution that worked.

Nonlinear thought helps you get beyond the conventional answers to find solutions. Rather than following the problem, you step away from the problem and look at the bigger picture.

## *Whole Brain Thinking*

As we said earlier, nearly everyone uses both the left and right sides of the brain. While one side usually dominates, it takes both to function appropriately and effectively. Whole-brain thinking is the process of consciously developing the nondominant aspect of your brain. Whole-brain thinkers can be simultaneously spontaneous and structured, logical and innovative, detail-oriented and visionary. They can see both the forest and the tree. While a few fortunate individuals are born whole-brained, most of us learn to develop a whole-brain approach to thinking and problem solving. The self-quiz earlier in this chapter gave you some insight on your brainedness. The following exercises can help you develop your nondominant brain side.

### Exercises to Improve Right Brain Functions

The right brain is free-flowing and creative. If you're left-brained, you might feel out of control in right-brain mode. Don't worry—you're not. You're just redefining control. To exercise your right brain, try these activities:

➤ Get in your car and drive off without any idea of where you're going or how long you'll be gone.

➤ Fly a kite.

➤ Prepare a favorite recipe from memory.

➤ Lay in bed for 10 minutes after your alarm goes off, and just let your mind wander.

➤ Paint with watercolors.

➤ Run or ride a bicycle (wear your helmet!) as fast as you can.

➤ Talk to yourself—out loud.

### Exercises to Improve Left Brain Functions

The left brain is structured and organized. If you're right-brained, you might feel stifled in left-brain mode. But you're not tied up. You're just giving order to your thoughts and actions.

➤ Put your music CDs in alphabetical order by artist.

➤ Play chess or checkers.

➤ Write out a plan for how you'll spend your time today.

➤ Follow the directions to assemble a piece of furniture.

➤ Match and fold your socks.

➤ Plan a trip by car, and then follow your plan.

➤ Organize your photographs into albums.

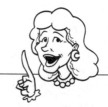

**Wise Woman's Wisdom**

"Learn to get in touch with the silence within yourself. There is no need to go to India or some-place else to find peace. You will find it in your room, your garden, or even your bathtub."

—Elisabeth Kübler-Ross

## Ambiguity and "Fuzzy" Thinking

Many people are uncomfortable with ambiguity. We like for there to be one way, one path, one answer. We believe that thinking should be a clear and orderly process, not a fuzzy and obscure jumble of mental meanderings. Ambiguity, it has been said, is much like herding cats: You can try to force order, but it's much easier to go with the flow. Fuzzy thinking, letting the edges blur as you attempt to solve a problem or find an answer, sometimes leads to incredible clarity in the form of a solution that wouldn't have occurred to your organized (left) brain.

# Embracing Intuition

You've heard it dozens of times: "It's just woman's intuition." *Just,* as if to dismiss or at least minimize the value. Intuition is a gift from your right brain, allowing you to receive and process information without going through the usual channels your left brain likes to use. But intuition is more like peripheral vision. It hovers around the edges of your conscious awareness, seeing what your brain hasn't yet detected.

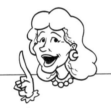

**Wise Woman's Wisdom**

"There is inside each of us a sixth sense: a soul sense which sees, hears, and feels all at the same time."

—Helen Keller

## Learning to Trust Your Wise Woman Hunches

Intuition may not be as mysterious as it appears. Although we perceive hunches as coming from nowhere, often they reflect the ability of your brain to collect and process thousands of tidbits of information without your conscious awareness. Rather than being based on some intangible and inexplicable signal, hunches may reflect your brain's ability to assimilate facts and observations at a speed much faster than you can think about them. People who can trust and act on their hunches often come up with great ideas and innovations.

## Tuning In to Your Wise Woman Senses

Everyone has intuition. It just takes practice to use it, especially if you're accustomed to disregarding or ignoring it. Perhaps you hear a tone in someone's voice that speaks volumes about how upset the person feels, even though his or her words give no hint of any distress. Maybe your sense of smell detects minute traces of smoke in the air, sending signals of danger throughout your body.

At one point in human development, our physical senses were far more refined than they are in our modern world. It's entirely likely that early humans could hear, smell, and possibly see with the sensitivity many animals have today. As the tools of civilization made life easier and safer, this sensitivity faded—the "use it or lose it" principle.

Is what we today call intuition a rebirth of this primal sensory sensitivity? It could be. If intuition seems, well, counterintuitive to you, try keeping a log of your intuitive experiences. Write down your hunches—what you feel, how you respond, and what happens. You might be surprised to discover that your inner senses are stronger and more accurate than you thought possible!

---

### The Least You Need to Know

➤ Most people have a dominant pattern of thinking and problem solving, either left brain or right brain.

➤ Understanding your dominant pattern can help you understand and relate to others.

➤ Developing your nondominant brain improves your ability to think and to solve problems.

➤ Estrogen seems to act as a chemical messenger in your brain that can expedite functions of memory and cognition.

➤ Estrogen therapy might be one way to prevent or delay memory loss and Alzheimer's disease.

➤ Intuition is your brain at work assimilating the myriad of information that your senses gather.

---

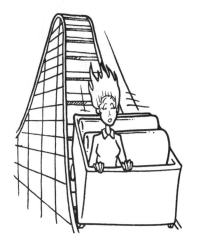

# Chapter 11

# Take a Ride on the Wild Side: Mood Swings

## In This Chapter

➤ How menopause affects your emotions

➤ How to know when the blues become depression

➤ How to identify and reduce stress in your life

➤ Learning to lighten your load and lean on your friends and family for support

➤ Reducing stress through exercise and meditation

➤ Menopause, too, shall pass

For some women, menopause is no different emotionally than any other time in their lives. There are good times and bad times, ups and downs, pleasures and griefs. These women may embrace menopause as a freedom train of sorts, transporting them from worries about pregnancy and the inconvenience of monthly periods to a new chapter in their lives.

For other women, the ride is bumpy. These women turn into personalities that are foreign even to themselves. They redefine the concept of mood swings as they vacillate, seemingly by the minute, between euphoria and despair. They don't sleep for weeks, and then can't stay awake for days. If this is a freedom train, they'd rather be slaves.

For most women, though, the menopause experience lies somewhere between—and sometimes touches—these two extremes. It might even be sometimes one, then the other. Menopause can be a wild ride!

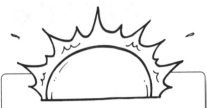

**Embracing Change**

When it comes to sleep, quality matters more than quantity. When hot flashes and other disturbances interrupt your sleep night after night, you can feel tired and tense. Try relaxation methods and calming techniques to help settle yourself down after you've been awakened. If you can get enough periods of deep sleep in which you enter a dream state, you'll feel more rested in the morning.

# I Love You So Much ... Go Away and Leave Me Alone!

The key aspect of mood swings is their absolute unpredictability. You can go from laughter to tears, joy to sorrow, nurture to anger in less time than it takes to finish a sentence. Often these conflicting emotions exist simultaneously, each demanding equal attention. It all leaves you feeling pulled and pushed and tugged and frayed. At the same time that you want others to love you, support you, and be there for you, you want to flee to a deserted island. There's nothing straightforward about this menopause journey.

## The Roller Coaster of Your Emotions

If PMS has been a companion through your fertile years, you already know that hormone fluctuations can produce quite a roller-coaster ride of emotions. First you're up, then suddenly you're down—and then you're back up again. While the ups are fine, those downs can be downright distressing—for you as well as for those around you. While hormones bear the brunt of blame for this wild ride, their involvement might be less direct than we've believed. Many experts believe that the signs of menopause create the problems, not hormone fluctuations. Hot flashes, for example, often interfere with sleep, as do irritation and stress. When your sleep cycle is constantly interrupted, your body fails to get the rest it needs. This leaves you feeling cranky and irritable, even if you think you're sleeping well.

## Coping with the Extremes

Mood swings, even wild ones, are a common accompaniment to menopause. For most women and the people in their lives, they're annoying but tolerable and transient. Hormone therapy, such as birth control pills or HRT, can provide relief for mood swings that are driven by fluctuating estrogen levels. Many women also find relief through dietary supplements high in phytoestrogens and herbal remedies (there's more discussion of this in Part 4, "HRT or No HRT, That Is the Question," and Part 5, "Menopause Treatment *Au Naturel*"). Exercise is a good way to burn off some of the day's stress, which can take the edge off the extremes of your mood swings. It also helps your body unwind and relax, better preparing it for more restful sleep.

## How to Know When You Need Help

If other people in your life get that deer-in-the-headlights look when they see you coming, your mood swings might be more than you can manage without some help from your doctor. Do you find yourself angry more often than not, or sad or anxious or listless? These could be signs of problems that need medical treatment, such as depression (more on this a little later in the chapter). Medical conditions such as hypothyroidism also can cause mood swings and other signs typically associated with menopause. If your mood swings are making life miserable for you or for those around you, see your doctor. This will let you eliminate other possible causes and help you make decisions about how best to moderate the effects of mood swings as you complete your transition through menopause.

# Are Your Slowing Hormones Dragging You Down?

During menopause, it may seem that your body is betraying you just when you need its resources the most. Your high-energy life runs out of steam. For reasons you can't explain through external events, you feel like you're running in slow motion. Your mind and heart just aren't in your work, your family, or your friends. You struggle to muster enough enthusiasm to get out of bed in the morning, you drag yourself through your day, and you feel wiped out by the day's end. What's up with this? For many women, it's more a matter of what's down. Those dropping hormone levels can make you feel down and blue.

## The Season of SADness

Seasonal affective disorder (SAD) is a form of depression linked to the diminishing amount of natural light during the winter months. Many experts believe that this is because natural light helps regulate the pineal gland's production of melatonin, a hormone that causes drowsiness. In the cycle of nature, the pineal gland produces more melatonin when darkness falls, encouraging sleep at night. When the light of dawn breaks, the pineal gland reduces melatonin production. Bright natural light also appears to increase your body's production of serotonin, one of the neurotransmitters in your brain. People with depression often have low serotonin levels.

SAD is not necessarily related to menopause. However, the likelihood for developing SAD increases with age. This may result in SAD emerging

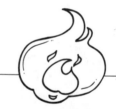

**Hot Flash!**

Tanning beds do *not* help with SAD. The ultraviolet lights of tanning beds are intended to stimulate skin cells to produce melanin, the substance that causes the skin's pigmentation to darken. These lights are harmful to the eyes (and to the skin).

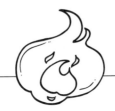

**Hot Flash!**

It can take as long as three months for antidepressant drugs to reign in the symptoms of depression. It is usually necessary to take these medications for six months to a year after your symptoms disappear. Interactions with other medications, including over-the-counter drugs, can cause serious problems. Always check with your doctor or pharmacist before taking any other drugs when you're taking an antidepressant.

**Wise Up**

**Serotonin** is a natural neurotransmitter found in the brain that is related to feelings of well-being as well as depression. **Melatonin** is a natural hormone that causes sleepiness.

at the same time a woman is entering menopause, giving the appearance of a connection. Because some of the signs of menopause are the same as the symptoms of SAD, women who have SAD often find that menopause makes their symptoms worse. Most people with SAD respond well to treatment with special lights designed to mimic the intensity and spectrum of natural sunlight.

## More Than the Blues: Depression

It's normal for everyone to feel down in the dumps now and then. Things happen that make us sad or angry or frustrated. Most of the time, we work through these feelings and return to our normal, cheerful selves. How long this takes depends on the individual and on the situation: Recovering from the death of a loved one may take several months to a year or longer, while getting over a reprimand by the boss may take until lunch. But when the stresses of life become overwhelming, or when deep sadness and hopelessness occur without apparent reason, the problem could be clinical depression, not just the blues.

Depression is a potentially serious medical condition that requires treatment. Although it's a common perception that menopause brings on increased rates of depression, studies fail to show a very distinctive correlation. Depression seems related to other biochemical functions, or malfunctions, in the brain. Often *serotonin* levels are low and *melatonin* levels are high in people suffering from clinical depression. The same correlation sometimes exists in women experiencing menopause, leading to interest in the relationship between estrogen and depression. So far, however, most studies show that depression is no more common among women at or beyond menopause than in women who are fertile.

Most experts agree that menopause does not cause depression. Certain events related to menopause can establish a setting that allows depression to more easily develop, however. Sleeping problems, for example, prevent your body and mind from getting needed rest and recovery from the stresses of everyday life. This can lead to the feelings of sadness and hopelessness that characterize depression. Treatment for depression aims at relieving the symptoms and addressing their underlying causes. In some situations, this involves restoring the brain's chemical balances through antidepressant medications such as Zoloft or Prozac, which increase serotonin levels in the brain. Some women prefer not to take antidepressant medications, instead finding relief through psychotherapy and behavioral therapy. And nonaddictive sleep aids can sometimes help provide enough relaxation to foster restful sleep. Be sure to use such products according to the label's instructions, and see your doctor if your sleep difficulties continue.

If you have any combination of the following signs of depression for more than two weeks, it's time to see your doctor or psychologist:

➤ Feelings of sadness, anxiety, emptiness, or hopelessness

➤ Problems going to sleep or staying asleep, or waking up early and being unable to go back to sleep

➤ Loss of interest in activities you used to enjoy

➤ Increased or decreased appetite

➤ Trouble remembering things, making decisions, or focusing

➤ Uncontrolled crying

➤ Irritability

➤ Thoughts of suicide or feelings that life isn't worth living

# Keeping a Handle on Stress

Everyone has stress in life. Without stress, of course, life would be nearly impossible. Stress gives you the boost you need to get things done. The problem is, for many people stress never goes away and becomes nonproductive. In the grand scheme of the human design, stress was intended to be a transitory experience, a cycle—a need generates pressure, action relieves the need, and the pressure goes away. That was the plan. What typically happens in today's world is that the third element in the cycle never happens. The stress stays high because a new need immediately replaces the satisfied need. Or, you aren't entirely able to satisfy the need, so it never quite goes away.

Recognition is a key aspect of controlling stress. One reason that stress controls your life is that you don't recognize the stress factors in your life. They have become so much a part of your daily existence that, like gray hair or wrinkles, you don't notice them until something forces a confrontation. The stress cycle is your mirror for these factors. Each time the stress cycle fails—you move right from one stress factor to another—this is like catching a glimpse of your gray hair as you pass by a reflective window. You don't have to do anything about your gray—and you might even wear it proudly. But each time you catch a glimpse of a stress factor, you have an opportunity to change it.

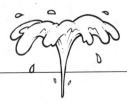

### Wellspring

Some studies suggest that medications used to treat depression, such as Prozac and Paxil, also relieve signs of menopause such as hot flashes in some women. Doctors aren't sure why this is, but they believe it has to do with the relationship between serotonin and estrogen. Antidepressants such as Prozac increase the levels of serotonin in the brain. Estrogen seems to act as a chemical facilitator, further smoothing communication among neurons (brain cells). While much study is still needed to explore these connections, this treatment approach holds promise for women who cannot take HRT, such as those who have had or are at high risk for breast cancer.

A challenge for many women is the tendency to take on more and more and more. This reflects a woman's nurturing nature, her desire and drive to care for and about the people who are important to her. This also generates unintended and often unobserved (dis)stress. Take a moment to think about everything that's on your mental to-do list right now. How much of it is for you, and how much of it is for others? This is not to say that doing for others is wrong or harmful. It's just a reminder to look at all that you do each day and see if it leaves you enough time and energy to care for and about you.

## Calling Timeout

A timeout is as useful for 50-year-olds as it is for 5-year-olds. The principle is the same: Put some distance between the source and the reaction. The only difference is that no one is going to put you on timeout—you'll need to do it yourself. Learn your warning signs and what stages of stress they signal. If you're not clear on this, ask a trusted friend to give you some honest feedback. It's hard to see yourself from the outside, as others see you. You'll need to learn to identify the outward signs from within so that you can intercept your responses before the situation becomes overwhelming.

## Lean on Your Support Network

This is a time to call on your friends and family for support and encouragement. Let those who are close to you know how you're feeling and what they can do to help. Communication is especially important because your mood swings and erratic behavior may have your loved ones wanting to help but uncertain about how to approach you. When you approach them, this makes it easier for them to know what to do and when to do it. This can be a difficult step if you, like many women, have always been the strong one, the one others turn to when they need support and help. But it's a necessary step—one attribute of strength is knowing when to call for reinforcements.

## Lighten Your Load

If your work never seems to get done, maybe it's time to examine your load. Just because you *can* multitask doesn't mean that you have to or that you should. Many women pick up the pieces others drop—kids, spouses, co-workers—without passing off what's already on their plates. Remember right brain/left brain dominance discussed in the previous chapter? If you're right-brained—someone who thrives on ambiguity and innovation—you probably have too much to do and not enough time or energy to do it all. You can see the forest, but you come up short when it comes to seeing the trees.

Try a left-brain exercise (even if you are left-brained) to get a better look at the trees in your life's forest. Take out a piece of paper and a pen or pencil. Starting with when you get up in the morning, divide the paper into portions for each four-hour segment of your waking day. Write down everything—*everything*—that you typically do during each segment. For each item, write down how much time it takes to do if it's the only thing you do. When you're finished, add up all the times. Do you need 30 hours in your day to do everything on your list? If so, it's time to pare down!

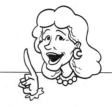

### Wise Woman's Wisdom

"It is my friends that have made the story of my life. In a thousand ways they have turned my limitations into beautiful privileges, and enabled me to walk serene and happy in the shadow cast by my deprivation."

—Helen Keller

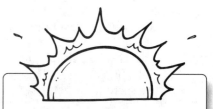

### Embracing Change

Many communities have support groups where people can share their experiences and concerns. Look in the Yellow Pages under "Support Groups," or search the Internet (enter keywords "support groups"). Local newspapers also often list the meeting times and locations of support groups.

Okay, so you find that you make your lists, cut them in half, and *still* try to do it all on your own? Try asking yourself some prioritizing questions. Answer honestly!

➤ Do you *enjoy* (yes, enjoy!) this task?

➤ Can someone else do this task as easily (or, if not as *easily*, then, as *effectively*) as you can?

➤ What is it about this task that you don't want to give up?

➤ Whose responsibility is this task *really*, anyway?

# Natural Ways to Reduce Stress

To reduce stress at the level of its causes, you first have to identify those causes. This can be a challenge because the stress is usually a cumulative process. It's not one isolated factor that stresses you, but multiple factors drawing on your resources and abilities all at the same time. As much as possible, lighten the load of your responsibilities. After you've done that, look for ways to improve your coping abilities in a general way.

## The Power of Exercise

Just as regular exercise can keep your body fit and toned, it also can keep your mind clear and focused. It's great if you can join a health club and get a structured, aerobically challenging workout three or four days a week. But even if you can't, a little bit of daily activity goes a long way. Just 30 minutes of walking three or four days a week is enough to lower blood pressure, lower blood levels of "bad" cholesterol and raise "good" cholesterol, and improve insulin sensitivity in most people. Vigorous exercise also releases natural chemicals in your body, called endorphins, that can make you feel a bit euphoric. This good feeling often extends for up to several hours following the exercise, which is a wonderful natural mood elevator.

Walking for 20 to 30 minutes at a stretch, at a moderately vigorous pace, is best. Even if your day is full, you can usually squeeze this in. Taking a brisk walk before lunch, for example, revitalizes your energy level and hikes your metabolism up a notch or two to burn more calories from your midday meal. If you feel that you can't squeeze 20 to 30 minutes out of your day for exercise, go for shorter segments and look for ways to be active in the course of your day. Take the stairs instead of the elevator. Park at the back of the lot or around the block, and walk to the office or store. A more leisurely walk in the evening can help you unwind and clear your mind before turning in for the night, helping you get a more restful night's sleep. Other activities such as tai chi, yoga, and martial arts can have the same benefits as conventional exercise.

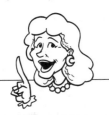

**Wise Woman's Wisdom**

"It's not the load that breaks you down. It's the way you carry it."

—Lena Horne

## Easing Your Cluttered Mind: Meditation

People who don't meditate often think of meditation as a process of clearing everything from their minds. The mere thought of this can be overwhelming enough to keep you from even trying meditation! There are many forms of meditation, however. The idea behind meditation is to retreat within yourself for a short time. Some people accomplish this by sitting outside, watching the clouds go by or listening to the birds in the trees. Others follow a more formalized process, retreating to a special place where they can sit in solitude and silence. Like exercise, meditation is most effective when you do it regularly.

## A 10-Minute Meditation Exercise

If meditation is new to you, try this exercise. Go to a place where you can be alone and uninterrupted for 10 minutes. It doesn't have to be any place special, although it often helps to get away from your daily environment by going outside or to another room. At first, use a timer or an alarm so that you meditate for exactly 10 minutes.

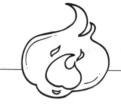

**Hot Flash!**

If you can't remember the last time you worked up a sweat, schedule a checkup with your doctor before embarking on an exercise plan. You might also want to have a fitness consultant help you design an exercise plan that can safely take you from where you are to where you want to be.

1. Sit down and get comfortable, and then start the timer.

2. Close your eyes. Take several slow, deep breaths. (Slow is the key here—fast deep breathing will cause you to hyperventilate and feel dizzy.)

3. Become aware of your thoughts. See them spinning and colliding through your mind. Are they fragments not connected to one another, or are they complete concepts?

4. Choose one thought and focus on it. Try to envision everything about it. Examine it with your mind as you might examine a strange object with your senses.

5. Let this single thought expand until it fills up your mind, crowding out all other thoughts. When other thoughts attempt to intrude, ignore them. Focus only on this single thought, and hold your focus for as long as you can.

6. When you become distracted or your timer goes off, release the thought slowly and gently, as you might release a butterfly. Let it return to its original size and state.

7. Notice what happens to the other thoughts that had been jumbled in your mind. Do they rush back in, or are they smaller and less significant, too?

8. Take several slow, deep breaths and open your eyes. You should feel refreshed and relaxed.

If you'd like to learn more about meditation and how you can use it to combat stress, you might enjoy *The Complete Idiot's Guide to Meditation* (Alpha Books, 1998).

# There's a Light at the End of the Tunnel, and It's *Not* a Train

It's important—and often difficult—to remember that menopause is a transition. It, and all its signs and challenges, will pass. Certainly, you will feel discouraged and overwhelmed on your journey; life has its ups and downs, and the transition of menopause is certainly no exception. Don't be afraid to ask for help from loved ones or from your doctor. While menopause is about change and challenge, it doesn't have to be about suffering. Many options are available to women today to ease the passage, and there's reason not to use them. Many women emerge from menopause feeling a confidence and strength that they didn't know they had. Like all life passages, menopause is about learning, changing, and growing. The more of its experiences you can embrace, the more positive your journey will be.

---

### The Least You Need to Know

➤ For some women, menopause is no different than any other time in their lives. For others, it is a wild ride on a roller coaster of emotions and feelings.

➤ Stress is a significant factor in feelings of hopelessness and despair. Reducing stress can improve these feelings.

➤ Many women need to learn how to lighten their loads to reduce stress and restore resources to themselves.

➤ No woman needs to suffer through menopause. Many options exist for relieving signs that cause discomfort.

➤ Remember that menopause is a transition, not a permanent state.

---

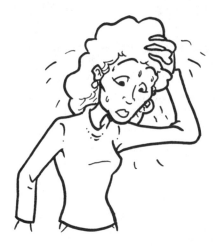

# Chapter 12

# Hot Flashes, Thinning Hair, and What's Happening *Down There*

## In This Chapter

➤ What causes hot flashes?

➤ How to manage hot flashes and chills

➤ How to get a more restful night's sleep

➤ When to worry about cancer

➤ What other changes take place in your body

An array of physical signs herald the approach of midlife. For many women, these signs are a wake-up call to pay attention to their bodies. They're telling you that this is a second spring, a time of renewal and opportunity. You have another chance to make healthy and positive changes to help shape the body that will carry you through the second half of your life.

The first sign strikes seemingly from nowhere. There you are, making a marketing presentation to a prospective client or enjoying a quiet evening at home when, whoom! A flood of heat surges through you, leaving your face and neck flushed. Perspiration drenches you. You look as though you've just stepped from a sauna. Everyone else, on the other hand, looks calm and cool, if not a bit puzzled by your sudden and apparent discomfort. Is it something you ate? The flu? A bizarre and deadly tropical disease that Aunt Rochelle brought back from her safari vacation? Nope. It's just a hot flash—and there are likely to be plenty more where that came from.

**Wise Up**

**Vasomotor regulation** is the process by which the body maintains a stable temperature. **Thermoregulatory dysfunction** is the technical term for the hot flashes and chills that often occur during menopause.

# Who Turned Up the Heat?

The hot flash is perhaps the most notorious and widely recognized announcement that menopause is underway. For reasons doctors don't fully understand, fluctuating estrogen levels interfere with your body's *vasomotor regulation*. Technically known as *thermoregulatory dysfunction,* a hot flash represents a momentary malfunction of your body's cooling mechanisms.

Dropping estrogen levels fool your body into acting as though it has become seriously overheated. It really hasn't, of course, although you suddenly feel very hot. But your vasomotor regulation process has already misinterpreted the signals, and its response is in full swing. The first line of reaction is dilation of the blood vessels near your skin's surface. Blood rushes into these vessels, causing your skin to flush. Because the blood is now closer to the outside, it cools. Then stage two hits: profuse sweating. Evaporating perspiration cools the skin, carrying away the heat brought to its surface.

Your body temperature hasn't really changed, so all this cooling is for naught. Sometimes the result is that as soon as the hot flash passes, you feel chilled. Hot flashes can last a brief 30 seconds or a seemingly eternal 2 to 3 minutes. The more drastic a woman's estrogen levels drop, the more severe her hot flashes tend to be. Women who enter menopause suddenly, such as those who have hysterectomies with the removal of ovaries, are often the most unfortunate in this regard. For more than half of the women who experience them, however, hot flashes are less extreme. Indeed, many women jokingly refer to them as power surges!

## Coping with Hot Flashes

For most women, hot flashes occur over a three- to five-year period of time when estrogen levels are most volatile. With rare exceptions, hot flashes end when menopause is complete. Whether you choose to put up with the inconvenience, try natural remedies, or seek medical treatment, you can take some basic steps to minimize the intrusion that hot flashes make into your life and everyday activities.

➤ Avoid potential trigger foods that can set off or intensify hot flashes. These include spicy foods, caffeine, and alcohol.

➤ Wear clothing made from natural fabrics. These items breathe, allowing heat and moisture to escape. They also absorb moisture when you perspire.

➤ Sleep on natural-fiber sheets. Put two sheets on your mattress, so you can peel one off if nighttime hot flashes cause enough sweating to dampen the sheet.

➤ Eat smaller, more frequent meals of nutritious foods to keep your blood insulin and sugar balance stable. There appears to be a correlation between insulin and estrogen.

➤ Let the little things go. Stress keeps your body in a state of alertness, which intensifies any experience it has. Reducing stress lets your body relax.

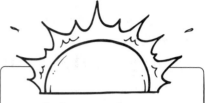

**Embracing Change**

Certain medications prescribed to treat depression appear to also reduce the frequency and severity of hot flashes, and your doctor might prescribe them to do so. These medications, such as Zoloft and Prozac, work by increasing the brain's serotonin levels. This seems to enhance the body's ability to produce estrogen, alleviating some of the signs of menopause.

## Medical Treatments

From a medical perspective, a single word summarizes the most effective treatment for hot flashes: estrogen. Not every woman who experiences hot flashes may need or desire estrogen replacement. For those who do, the typical choices are birth control pills (if premenopausal) or HRT. Natural micronized progesterone pills or vaginal cream can also help with hot flashes, and some women get relief from vitamin E supplements. Which is medically appropriate for you depends on your personal circumstances. These may include your age, how your hot flashes affect you, and whether you have a personal or family history of breast or uterine cancer. The chapters in Part 4, "HRT or No HRT, That Is the Question," provide a comprehensive discussion of estrogen replacement.

## Natural Remedies

A number of herbal remedies on the market claim to relieve hot flashes and other signs of menopause. Some work well for some women, especially those whose hot flashes are less severe. Natural remedies tend not to be as effective when estrogen fluctuations are dramatic, such as in surgical menopause. Foods containing soy have high amounts of substances called isoflavones. Isoflavones are phytoestrogens, estrogen hormones that come from plant sources. Isoflavones also lower blood cholesterol levels. Good sources of soy-based isoflavones are tofu, soy milk, soybeans, soynuts, and tempeh. Don't expect to get much relief from soy sauce, miso, or most soy burgers, though. These products are highly processed and retain very little in the way of isoflavones.

Herbal remedies are becoming increasingly popular. Many women experience relief from substances such as dong quai (a Chinese herb) and black cohosh (used by early Native Americans). These and other herbal remedies can interact with other medications you might be taking, though, so always check with your doctor before taking them. Chapter 19, "Soy, Herbs, and Other Botanicals: Nature's Menopause Miracles," discusses herbal and other natural remedies.

# Bring on the Flannel and the Blankets!

Not all flashes are hot. Some women experience severe chills following or even without hot flashes. The same physiological mechanisms—vasomotor regulation and thermoregulatory dysfunction—cause both hot flashes and cold chills. Instead of feeling a flood of heat rush through your body, you feel an intense chill. For its duration—which, like a hot flash, is typically 30 seconds to several minutes—there is no escaping it.

## *When Hot Flashes Turn to Chills*

For the woman who experiences raging hot flashes, chills might seem like heaven. But for the woman who has them, chills are no party. It's just as unpleasant (even if it's not as obvious to others) to be too cold as it is to be too hot. No matter how warm you try to get, you still feel chilled to the bone. Once the chill passes, your sense of temperature returns to normal.

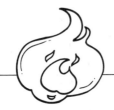

**Hot Flash!**

Because chills and feeling cold also can be symptoms of medical conditions such as hypothyroidism, it's important to have your doctor check you out before chalking these signs up to menopause. Hypothyroidism requires a different treatment.

## *Medical Treatments*

Because chills are the same type of thermoregulatory dysfunction as hot flashes, the same medical treatment options can help. Replacing the body's estrogen seems to restore thermal equilibrium, greatly reducing or even ending the seesaw ride of reactions. For many women, chills accompany hot flashes, so medical treatment covers both. Women who experience only chills may not recognize at first that chills, like hot flashes, are treatable signs of menopause.

## *Natural Remedies*

The same layering recommendations that are often effective for coping with hot flashes can help with chills. Instead of peeling off clothing, however, you'll be piling on the layers. Light, natural fabrics are most effective because they warm quickly when they come in contact with your skin. Drinking warm fluids, such as tea, can also help you feel warmer. If your chills happen in tandem with hot flashes, though, be careful about warming too much: Excess heat can trigger hot flashes.

Herbs and other natural remedies that relieve hot flashes generally work well for chills, too. The same cautions and warnings apply. Talk with your doctor before you start taking any natural remedy, just to be sure that it won't interact with a medication you're taking or cause other health problems for you. There's more on natural remedies in Chapter 19.

# Sleepless in Midlife

Sleep patterns often change during menopause. Many women find it difficult to fall asleep when they first go to bed, tossing and turning for several hours before finally drifting off. The sleep that results may also be restless, interrupted by periods of waking. Some women initially fall asleep with little difficulty but can't go back to sleep after waking up in the middle of the night. Hot flashes are often the culprit, rousing you partially or fully from sleep. When this happens, it interrupts your deep, or *REM,* sleep.

Although REM sleep is the shorter of the two kinds of sleep (the other is NREM, or nonrapid eye movement), it's the one that appears to be more important for restfulness. During REM sleep, your brain's electrical activity dramatically increases, and your eyes flutter and move rapidly behind your closed eyelids. REM sleep occupies a progressively longer share of each 90-minute sleep cycle, beginning with about 10 minutes of the first cycle after you fall asleep and concluding with nearly an hour of the last cycle before you wake up.

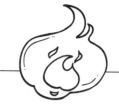

**Hot Flash!**

Over-the-counter sleeping products may do you more harm than good, leaving you feeling "hung over" and unrested the next day. If getting a good night's sleep has become mission impossible, see your doctor to check out the possible causes and discuss potential solutions.

**Wise Up**

**REM** stands for rapid eye movement and identifies the stage of sleep during which dreaming occurs.

Researchers don't fully understand the body's need for sleep, but dreaming seems to be a critical element of your brain's ability to rest and recharge itself. When REM sleep—dream sleep—is interrupted, you feel tired and sluggish the next day. The later into the sleep cycle interruptions take place, the more disruptive they are.

Hot flashes can interrupt sleep without fully awakening you. By morning, you don't remember that you suddenly kicked the covers off and thrashed around (although your partner might). But your body does, and you feel the effects. There are other reasons for why you might not be sleeping well during this transitional period in your life, too. Stress and tension can keep your mind active and awake when your body wants to be asleep. Try these tips to improve your odds for a more restful night's sleep:

➤ Get moderately intense physical exercise every day (but not right before you go to bed). This helps keep your cells and tissues operating at peak performance.

➤ Use stress-relief techniques such as focused imagery, meditation, or biofeedback to help you relax and get rid of the day's worries and problems.

➤ Reduce the amount of caffeine, fat, and sugar in your daily diet. Don't eat within an hour of going to bed.

➤ Go to bed and get up at the same time every day, regardless of whether you feel wide awake or sleepy.

➤ Shut the curtains or blinds and the door to keep your bedroom dark while you're sleeping, and to close out distracting sounds.

# AUB, DUB: When Is the Bleeding Too Much?

Sometimes vaginal bleeding during menopause is normal. HRT and birth control pills that include both estrogen and progesterone each restore your body's hormonal balance. Most treatment regimens deliver these hormones in a cycle that emulates your body's natural hormonal cycle. As a result, some women experience periodlike bleeding each month. Such bleeding is predictable and moderate, and may eventually go away as your body's natural hormone levels continue to change. This bleeding, called dysfunctional uterine bleeding (DUB), is most likely to disappear altogether when HRT is continuous (see Chapter 14, "What Is Hormone Replacement Therapy (HRT)?" for more information). Often your doctor can eliminate DUB by starting you on HRT or by modifying your HRT regimen.

Sometimes bleeding is heavy or wildly irregular, or starts again after months or years without bleeding. In these circumstances, have your doctor check you out. Although serious health problems such as cancer are relatively rare, their likelihood increases with age. Abnormal uterine bleeding (AUB) generally has a clinical reason. Perhaps there are uterine fibroids or other medical conditions. Because AUB can indicate a precancerous condition or cancer itself, medical evaluation and treatment is essential.

## Could It Be Cancer?

Vaginal bleeding can be a worrisome sign. Even though women bleed every month with their menstrual periods, bleeding is still an event that we tend to associate more with problems than with normal processes. This is particularly true when you think that your periods have stopped, and then all of a sudden you're bleeding again. It's natural to worry, because unexpected vaginal bleeding can be a sign of a serious health condition such as cancer, and that's a good reason to have your doctor check you over.

But most of the time, this bleeding is not serious. Other growths in the uterus, such as *polyps* and *fibroids*, can cause bleeding. Doctors often recommend surgery to remove these growths, which can have the potential to become cancerous.

Because cancer is always a possibility, you should notify your doctor about any unusual or unexpected bleeding. Doctors consider vaginal bleeding abnormal under these circumstances:

➤ It saturates more than one pad or tampon an hour for more than eight hours.

➤ Pain accompanies the bleeding.

➤ Bleeding starts for no apparent reason or doesn't seem cyclical.

➤ It has been several to many years since you passed menopause (had your last menstrual period).

**Wise Up**

A **polyp** is an abnormal growth that usually forms in mucous membrane tissue such as the cervix. A **fibroid** is a growth of muscle and connective tissue that forms in the uterus.

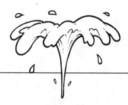

**Wellspring**

More than 14,000 women are diagnosed with invasive cervical cancer each year, and nearly 5,000 women will die from it. The good news is that doctors now know what causes nearly all cervical cancer: a virus called human papillomavirus (HPV). This virus shows up in 60 or so variations, several of which are linked to cervical and vaginal cancers; one variation causes genital warts. HPV can lurk in the body for years without causing any symptoms, and then emerge as cancer. Regular Pap tests and pelvic exams are an easy way to detect changes in cervical cells at an early stage, improving the odds that treatment will cure the cancer.

## Narrowing the Possibilities

The first step in determining whether bleeding is abnormal or dysfunctional is a physical exam, including a careful history. Expect your doctor to do a thorough pelvic exam and Pap smear, and to ask questions about your menstrual pattern through your reproductive years, your sexual activity, and the history of your current symptoms. It's important for your responses to be as specific as possible. This helps to zero in on the underlying cause of the bleeding. Depending on the initial findings, your doctor might want further tests. These might include blood tests, an ultrasound, or a *hysteroscopy*.

**Wise Up**

A **hysteroscopy** is a procedure during which the doctor passes a lighted magnifying scope through the vagina and cervix into the uterus to look for abnormalities. Hysteroscopy can often be done in the doctor's office.

## Choosing Appropriate Treatments

Of course, treatment depends on the diagnosis. Although cancer is relatively uncommon compared to the range of diagnostic findings, it generally requires immediate treatment to remove the cancerous tissue. This might include laser surgery or cryosurgery to superheat or superfreeze the cancerous cells, or hysterectomy. More advanced cancers require a more aggressive approach that includes some combination of surgery, radiation therapy, and chemotherapy.

The majority of unusual bleeding is dysfunctional uterine bleeding (DUB). Your body is experiencing a kind of withdrawal from estrogen and progesterone as your levels of these hormones drop. Medical interventions such as HRT or birth control pills often help, although these are not necessary if your doctor has eliminated any underlying problems and you're willing to put up with the bleeding for what is usually no longer than a year or two. For most women who experience it, DUB goes away at the completion of menopause.

**Wise Up**

**Iron deficiency anemia** is a health condition in which the blood's red cells are low in hemoglobin, reducing their ability to carry oxygen.

## Living with DUB

As a manifestation of menopause, DUB can certainly be frustratingly inconvenient. Although the bleeding is typically light, its irregularity makes it difficult for you to be prepared. Many women find some relief through herbal and natural menopause remedies that boost estrogen levels, such as dong quai and black cohosh. Regular exercise and a nutritional diet also help your body regain its rhythm. Some women worry about *iron deficiency anemia* resulting from the bleeding. This is something that your doctor will monitor through blood tests, but anemia isn't as common during menopause as during the years of menstruation because blood loss is much less. Be sure to have your doctor check your blood hemoglobin level before you take an iron supplement. Too much iron is a serious health problem, and it doesn't take much to get to that point.

# What's Happening to Your Body?

For most of your adult life, your hormones have functioned in the background. You become aware of them every month, of course, but only to the extent that they caused your periods. Menopause is like a window looking in on the full picture of the role your hormones play in how your entire body functions. As estrogen and progesterone levels retreat, not only do your periods stop, but a series of other physical changes also take place. Body fat distribution patterns change—what once settled on your hips and thighs now takes up residence across your middle, wanting to form a belly paunch. Your hair thins, loses color, and becomes brittle. The natural lubrication keeping your vaginal tissues moist diminishes, and the tissues become thinner. But it's not as bad as it might sound. There are a number of actions you can take to reduce the effects that these changes have.

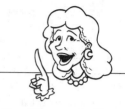

**Wise Woman's Wisdom**

"I have everything now I had 20 years ago—except now it's all lower."

—Gypsy Rose Lee

**Embracing Change**

Those hairs you perceive as gray are actually devoid of any pigmentation, making them white. They appear gray, however, when mixed with your normally colored hair.

## What Your Hairdresser Won't Tell You

Those first few gray hairs didn't seem like such a big deal. You could pluck them out or bury them under the rest of your hair, and no one else was the wiser. (Contrary to the old wives' tale, you don't grow three new gray hairs to replace every one you pluck out!) But now gray is your predominant color, and your once silken locks have developed a texture better suited to rope. What gives? Well, your hair, actually. Your hair follicles lose their ability to regenerate lost hair and to produce pigmentation.

Gradual hair loss does continue as you grow older, although for most women this does not become a problem. Many products on the market today enhance your hair's body and fullness. If you've colored your hair when its pigmentation was normal, you'll notice the changes in pigmentation. Your hairdresser can help you select colors and products specially designed to cover gray.

## *Vaginal Dryness and Itching*

Dropping estrogen levels alter the elasticity and lubrication in vaginal tissues. This can result in dryness, itching, and discomfort during sexual intercourse. For most women, these signs, like hot flashes and mood swings, disappear once menopause is complete. Prescription vaginal creams containing estrogen are often helpful in the interim (but don't apply such a product just before sex, as it can affect the man). Some women also get relief from vaginal vitamin E or aloe vera products that are available without a prescription. Water-based lubricants can significantly reduce any discomfort during sexual intercourse. The old adage "use it or lose it" gains new meaning at menopause. Regular sex is one of the most effective ways to improve vaginal lubrication and tissue vitality, not just during intercourse, but overall as well.

# Making Peace with Your Changing Body

The physical changes of menopause can be disconcerting to those who are not expecting them or who don't understand why they happen. But your body has been changing all your life. Life, in fact, is change. True, you won't again have the body of a 25-year-old. But you do have the grace and wisdom that comes with experience and maturity. Menopause is a great time to become reacquainted with your body, if you've drifted away from conscious awareness of its presence and functions. And it's an opportunity to marvel at the wonder of the body that gives you life. Even in its changing form, it is truly a beautiful and amazing creation.

---

### **The Least You Need to Know**

➤ Hot flashes, cold chills, and withdrawal bleeding are common during menopause and usually go away when the menopause transition is complete.

➤ Estrogen supplementation is the most effective medical treatment for reducing the discomforts of many menopause signs. Many women can use natural supplements such as herbs and food-based products.

➤ Your doctor should check out any unusual vaginal bleeding to eliminate serious health conditions such as cancer.

➤ Regular sex is the most effective way to restore your body's natural vaginal lubrication and tissue vitality.

---

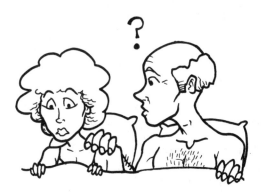

# Chapter 13

# Sexuality, Those 10 Extra Pounds, and Menopause

## In This Chapter

➤ How "male" hormones affect your sexuality

➤ How to overcome discomfort during sex

➤ How to manage your body's metabolic changes

➤ A self-quiz: How fat-savvy are you?

➤ Understanding and communicating your needs

➤ Feeling good about yourself in this time of change

Menopause is a time of challenge when it comes to your changing sense of your sexuality. Even if you spent most of your childbearing years avoiding pregnancy, your fertility has been the essence of your femininity. In fact, the word *feminine* has its origins in the Latin word *fecundus,* which means "to be fruitful." Fecundity, or the ability to become pregnant, ends with menopause.

Does this mean that femininity ends with menopause, too? Not by any stretch of the imagination! Menopause may redefine femininity, but by no means does it make you any less of a woman than you've always been. In many ways, it makes you more of a woman than you've ever been.

# Losin' That Lovin' Feeling

Menopause initiates a change in sex drive for many women. From a purely biological perspective, it makes perfect sense for a woman in midlife to lose interest in sex. After all, she's not going to be making any more babies. Her *body* doesn't know about the many ways to prevent pregnancy, so it does what it can—it shuts down her sexual drive. But humans are not pure biology. We are thoughtful, caring, social beings. We need and want loving relationships for the intimacy and connectedness they offer, not just for the biological purpose of reproduction.

## Wise Up

**Androgens** are the hormones responsible for secondary sex characteristics in men and libido in both genders. **Libido** is a person's sex drive or interest in sexual activity.

## Androgens and Sex Drive

While estrogen takes the heat for most of the changes associated with menopause, the focus shifts to *androgens* when it comes to *libido*. We generally think of androgens as the "male" hormones, but the bodies of both men and women produce androgens (as well as what we think of as the "female" hormones, the estrogens). The most common and familiar androgen in both male and female bodies is testosterone. In the male body, this is the hormone responsible for secondary sex characteristics such as facial and body hair. The male sex glands, the testes (also called testicles), produce most of a man's testosterone. His adrenal glands produce smaller amounts of testosterone and other androgens, as well as minute amounts of estrogens. (Researchers don't fully understand the role of estrogen hormones in the male body.)

In the female body, the ovaries and adrenal glands produce very small amounts of androgens, predominantly androstenedione and testosterone. Androstenedione is called an estrogen precursor—from it, a woman's body makes estrogen. Estrogen—more specifically, the estrogen hormone estrodiol—stimulates androgen production. So, there's a tight circle connecting these hormones in a woman's body. When one changes—for example, estrogen production declines as follicle activity diminishes—it affects the others.

At menopause, a woman's testosterone level drops by half or more. Many doctors believe that this is responsible for signs such as lack of interest in sex and perpetual tiredness or fatigue. When a woman's testosterone levels are low, HRT that includes a tiny amount of testosterone supplement can often help. Some research suggests that testosterone supplementation aids estrogen in building bone and reducing the risk of osteoporosis.

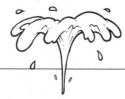

### Wellspring

In the human body, testosterone exists in two forms: free and bound. Both are important when trying to determine whether low testosterone is responsible for a woman's low libido and other problems. Most of the testosterone is bound, or attached to proteins in the blood. The testosterone that's not bound is free and is the testosterone that influences a woman's sex drive and energy levels. Blood tests to measure testosterone can measure total testosterone and free testosterone. It's possible (and surprisingly common) for a woman's total testosterone level to be normal and her free testosterone level to be low, causing symptoms.

## Other Hormonal Influences

Changing estrogen and progesterone levels cause changes in vaginal tissues and lubrication that can make sex suddenly and markedly less enjoyable—and even painful. The body's natural secretions become less abundant, and a woman's genitalia can feel dry and irritated. Sexual arousal can take longer, too. Over time, vaginal tissues can become thinner and less resilient as well. At the risk of sounding crass, the best cure for these changes is frequent use! Women who engage in sexual activity (including masturbation) often and regularly are far less likely to experience drastic changes in vaginal tissues.

## Viagra for Women?

When Viagra (a brand name for the impotency drug sildenafil) hit the market in the late 1990s, millions of men with erectile difficulties swamped doctors' offices with requests for this miracle in a little blue pill. Viagra increases a man's ability to get and maintain an erection. To understand how Viagra works, you need to understand how an erection happens.

When a man becomes aroused, smooth muscle tissues such as those in the walls of the penis produce the chemical nitric oxide. The increased level of nitric oxide causes the release of another chemical called cyclic GMP. Cyclic GMP allows the muscles in the penis to relax so that the erectile tissues can fill with blood. This causes the penis to become enlarged and firm. Because a permanent erection is much less desirable than it might sound (without fresh blood to bring oxygen, the tissues would die), the man's body also produces a chemical called PDE5. PDE5's mission is to

**137**

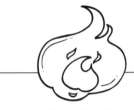

### Hot Flash!

People who are taking nitrate-based medications commonly prescribed for heart conditions such as angina should *not* take Viagra or similar products. Taking two nitrate-based drugs at the same time can cause the blood vessels to dilate throughout the body, resulting in a sudden drop in blood pressure.

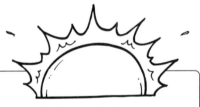

### Embracing Change

Is your relationship struggling? Midlife is a challenging time for many reasons. A therapist who specializes in relationship issues can help you sort through your feelings, worries, and concerns. Your regular doctor or health clinic can refer you to a therapist who is qualified and appropriately licensed.

counteract nitric oxide to reduce the flow of cyclic GMP. As cyclic GMP drops, so does the erection. Viagra works by slowing the production of PDE5. Less PDE5 means that the level of nitric oxide stays higher for longer, and so the penis stays firmer for longer.

Very interesting, but just what does this have to do with women, you ask? Well, the tissues of the clitoris are the same tissues as those of the penis. While there haven't yet been extensive tests of Viagra use in women, there is considerable speculation that what's good for the gander is also good for the goose. A few small studies have shown that Viagra does in fact have the same effect on the clitoris and the walls of the vagina as it does on the penis: increased blood engorgement. This appears to heighten sensitivity, making sex more pleasurable and enabling women to more easily achieve orgasm. As of this book's writing, however, Viagra (which requires a doctor's prescription) is not approved for women to use.

## Beyond Hormones

Decreasing hormones aren't always to blame for diminishing libido. Sometimes issues within a relationship interfere with sex drive. It's difficult to feel romantic when financial or career challenges preoccupy your thoughts. Some couples lose sight of what holds them together during the years when raising children takes over their lives, and then they don't know how to relate to one another when the kids leave home. Some partners haven't really gotten along for quite some time, but they have been able to hide from the reality until their relationship confronts a life junction such as menopause.

Beyond its role in reproduction, sex is the most intimate communication between two partners. When the elements of intimacy are lacking, interest in sex often drops off. Menopause, as a time of life when it's natural to reflect and evaluate your life, can also be a time when intimacy issues come to the surface.

Lack of interest in making love reflects these struggles more so than sex drive (hormones). If your interest in sex seems low and your doctor can't find a physical reason, or if medical therapies such as HRT don't help, consider seeking advice from a couples' therapist. This can focus a more objective spotlight on your concerns and feelings.

# What Used to Be Fun Isn't Anymore

As your body changes in midlife, so does the way it functions and feels. Your needs and interests change, too. You may find that sexual activities you once enjoyed no longer give you the same pleasures. Some of this has nothing to do with your changing body, of course. It's natural for interests and desires to grow and change with maturity and experience. Many women find midlife to be a time of reconsidering many dimensions of their lives. Sometimes, however, the physical changes of menopause do affect sexual activity. Attempts to arouse can instead irritate tender tissues.

## Sex and Your Body's Changes

Many of menopause's physical changes take place gradually. While this is good in the sense that it gives your body—and your mind—time to adapt and adjust, it can create a challenge when it comes to recognizing why things are suddenly different when it comes to sex. The longer-term effects of lowered estrogen and progesterone levels, which also progress over time, include shortening of the vaginal channel. This can require changes in the angle and depth of penetration during intercourse. These are not insurmountable problems, by any means, but you must recognize the potential for them to be present so that you can take steps to minimize their effects. Many women find that once they free their minds and imaginations to envision sex differently, the changes of menopause bring about positive changes in their sex lives.

## Sex After Hysterectomy

Most women who have hysterectomies have few sexual difficulties after the incision heals. To an extent, this depends on the reason for the hysterectomy. Conditions such as cancer may involve more extensive surgery and continued treatment. The majority of hysterectomies are performed for other reasons, such as fibroids and dysfunctional bleeding. Particularly if you've had years of health problems and treatment efforts before your hysterectomy, life after surgery can feel blessedly free. Any pain or bleeding is usually gone, and so are concerns about contraception.

Some women do have problems such as vaginal dryness and difficulty becoming aroused or reaching orgasm following hysterectomy. Doctors believe that the cause might be the interruption of nerves and tiny blood vessels that occurs during surgery. More extended lovemaking, with a focus on foreplay to reach complete arousal before penetration and additional lubrication, can sometimes overcome this.

## If Sex Becomes Uncomfortable or Painful

Your body's changes can sometimes cause sex to become uncomfortable or even painful. At times even attempts at arousal are more of a turn-off than a turn-on. Such difficulties often stem from the reduction in natural moisture in your vaginal tissues. These tissues can be more tender than they used to be and may need gentle but extended stimulation. And sometimes penetration is painful because you're not fully aroused.

Sex should be fun and pleasurable. If it's not, schedule a checkup with your woman's healthcare specialist. Your healthcare provider can be sure that there aren't any physical problems that need attention. This is a good time to discuss hormone replacement options as well. If you're already taking HRT, birth control pills, or natural supplements, your doctor might want to alter your regimen or add a testosterone supplement.

Be sure to involve your partner in your search for solutions. It often helps to talk about what feels good and what doesn't. Be gentle, and take a positive attitude. This isn't a process of complaint or criticism, but a healthy and affirming discussion about how to improve the joys of lovemaking for both of you as your lives and your relationship evolve to the next level.

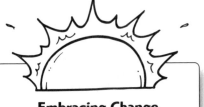

### Embracing Change

Some women find that they gain weight when they start HRT. While weight gain is a common side effect of various hormone use, including birth control pills, some studies suggest that weight gain associated with HRT is actually the weight gain that tends to occur with menopause.

## Adapting Can Be Fun

Look at this junction in your life and the changes it's thrusting at you as a time to try new adventures! This is the ideal opportunity to evaluate what you like—and what you'd like to try. It's a time to break free of habits that have developed out of routine, or because sex has long been something you've had to squeeze into an otherwise hectic schedule. It isn't always easy to shift from quickies to extended lovemaking, but it can be well worth the effort.

## When the Scale Betrays You

Once upon a time, all it took to get rid of that extra winter weight was a spring of extra exercise. If it seems that now even remembering those holiday goodies rolls up the numbers on the scale, it's not just your imagination. With increasing age comes decreasing metabolism. A 45-year-old woman needs about 150 fewer calories per day to meet her body's nutritional needs than a 25-year-old woman. That might not sound like that much, but it translates into about a pound a month.

# Is Weight Gain Inevitable?

Nearly all women gain a certain amount of weight as they pass through menopause, typically about 15 pounds between ages 30 and 60. No single reason accounts for this, although shifts in metabolism as a result of hormone changes play a major role. To compound the situation, your body shifts the ways and places it carries extra weight. What once settled around your hips and thighs now wants to nestle around your middle. Regular exercise and nutritious eating habits can help you keep the extra calories to a minimum, although the tendency for the ones you do collect to gather at your midsection is irresistible. Body proportions also change, with the pelvis widening and the shoulders narrowing. This can give the impression of a spreading waistline, even if you don't have one.

The Western culture's adoration of the super-thin supermodel leads women to believe that fat is bad. True, some health risks are associated with obesity, including heart disease, high blood pressure, and diabetes. But most doctors agree that an obsession with thinness is far more detrimental than gaining a few pounds. Rather than anguishing over that extra weight that just won't go away, you'll be happier if you can appreciate the body that you had when you were 25 years old as a fond memory and then accept the body that you have at age 50 as a comfortable and familiar friend—it's a friend that you need to treat with kindness and care, of course, but it's still a beloved friend. Worry less about fitting into your old clothes and more about staying fit!

**Embracing Change**

Does extra body fat protect you from hot flashes and other signs of menopause? A woman's fat cells do produce small amounts of estrogen, and some evidence indicates that women who have an abundant supply of fat cells have less significant signs of menopause than their fat-challenged counterparts. But don't rush out to pack on the pounds. The estrogen boost isn't worth the trade-off in increased health risks.

# Metabolic Changes

Muscle mass begins diminishing around age 35 to 40, and fat cells move in to fill the gap. At the same time, your metabolism begins to slow, so it takes fewer calories to meet your body's energy needs. In its endless preparations for the likelihood that you could face an extended time with little or no food (a vestige of primal existence when food was abundant in summer and scarce in winter), your body converts calories it doesn't need into—you guessed it—fat cells. And as your metabolism slows down, it becomes less efficient. Your cells become more resistant to insulin, causing your body to produce more of this vital hormone to do the same job. The older you get, the less your body is able to extract the vitamins and minerals from the foods you eat.

## *Healthy Eating to Support the New You*

Now is a great time to evaluate your eating habits. Try eating smaller amounts more frequently, and eat only until you feel full. Increase the fresh vegetables and fruits in your diet, and cut back on fats, carbohydrates, and sugars. The American Heart Association recommends that your fat calories account for 30 percent or less of your daily intake. The average American diet contains about 40 percent fat, well above the recommendation. Because a woman's risk for heart disease increases after menopause as she loses the protective benefits of estrogen, it's especially important to eat nutritiously. Most women benefit from increasing the phytoestrogens (soy) and omega-3 fatty acids (flaxseed) in their diets.

As your metabolism slows, your daily calorie needs decrease by 10 to 20 percent. However, eating is a habit, and old habits die hard. We eat because it's mealtime, because we're under stress, or because someone else is eating. Occasionally we eat because we're hungry, although we seldom stop when we're full (unless that coincides with an empty plate). At best, daily calorie intake remains the same—and may increase without conscious awareness that it's happening.

*Take a look at the nutrition guidelines in the USDA Food Guide Pyramid.*

# Food Guide Pyramid
## A Guide to Daily Food Choices

Fats, Oils, & Sweets
**USE SPARINGLY**

KEY
☐ Fat (naturally occurring and added)   ▪ Sugars (added)
These symbols show that fat and added sugars come mostly from fats, oils, and sweets, but can be part of or added to foods from the other food groups as well.

Milk, Yogurt, & Cheese Group
**2-3 SERVINGS**

Meat, Poultry, Fish, Dry Beans, Eggs, & Nuts Group
**2-3 SERVINGS**

Vegetable Group
**3-5 SERVINGS**

Fruit Group
**2-4 SERVINGS**

Bread, Cereal, Rice, & Pasta Group
**6-11 SERVINGS**

SOURCE: U.S. Department of Agriculture/U.S. Department of Health and Human Services

142

# A Self-Quiz: Where's the Fat?

Even when you're watching your fat intake, sometimes it's hard to know what the healthier option is when weighing menu selections. Try your hand at these choices to see how fat-savvy you are. From each pairing, choose the food that's lower in fat:

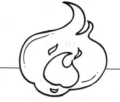

1. A super-sized order of McDonald's French fries, or a taco salad from Taco Bell?

2. A bagel with cream cheese, or a cheeseburger?

3. A roast beef sandwich or a tuna salad sandwich?

4. Broiled chicken breast or broiled salmon?

5. A milk chocolate candy bar or a piece of chocolate fudge?

6. A bowl of granola or a doughnut?

7. Two slices of bacon or two eggs?

8. A glass of milk or a bottle of beer?

9. A baked potato or homestyle fries?

10. A 12-ounce portion of filet mignon or a 12-ounce lobster tail?

**Hot Flash!**

Low-fat doesn't always mean low-calorie. For example, a half-cup of low-fat ice cream contains just 1 gram of fat compared to 12 grams of fat in regular ice cream. But the low-fat version has only 40 fewer calories—140 compared to 180. Read product labels carefully to compare.

Let's see how well you did. Here are the answers:

1. The fries are the better choice, although you wouldn't want to make either of these fast food items a staple in your diet. A super-sized order of McDonald's French fries contains 26 grams of fat, 4.5 grams of which are saturated. The Taco Bell taco salad has twice as much total fat and three times as much saturated fat: 52 grams of total fat, 15 grams of which are saturated. This salad's generous portions of cheese, beef, and dressing give it a whopping 840 calories.

2. Go with the burger, but hold the mayo. More than 90 percent of cream cheese's calories come from fat, compared to less than a third of that for extra-lean ground beef and low-fat cheese. Ketchup, mustard, and pickle relish are good no-fat condiment choices, but mayonnaise gets all of its 100 calories per tablespoon from fat.

3. Lean roast beef wins, hands down. Again, mayonnaise is the culprit. You're likely to get more mayo in a typical tuna salad sandwich than if you had mayo on your roast beef sandwich. And tuna packed in oil can have more fat than lean roast beef, which gets about 10 percent of its calories from fat.

4. The better choice comes down to the skin with these options. Chicken breast broiled with the skin and broiled salmon get about 25 percent of their calories from fat. Skin that chicken breast before cooking, however, and you drop nearly half its fat calories.

5. Fudge lovers, rejoice! This decadently delicious treat gets 18 percent of its calories from fat (35 percent of them saturated). Fat accounts for twice as many of the calories in milk chocolate, on the other hand (85 percent of them saturated).

6. These could be a draw, depending on how you eat them. A plain cake doughnut gets 25 percent of its calories from fat, with granola typically weighing in at about 20 percent (although some brands are significantly higher in fat). Frostings and fillings boost the doughnut's fat content, just as whole milk boosts the fat content of a bowl of granola.

7. Bacon might have a bad reputation, but it's the better choice when it comes to fat. Eggs get an incredible 80 percent of their calories from fat, compared to bacon's 23 percent. The fat content of those eggs jumps even higher when they're fried.

**Embracing Change**

Do you need to lose a few extra pounds? Try cutting 500 calories from your diet each day. In seven days, this adds up to 3,500 calories, the number of calories in a pound of fat. Add in 30 minutes of exercise each day to increase your metabolism, and you'll burn even more calories.

8. Beer contains no fat, although it also has no nutritional value and its carbohydrate calories can quickly turn to body fat. Whole milk has 8 grams of fat per cup, along with a number of important nutrients, including calcium and vitamin D. Skim milk, with less than a half-gram of fat, contains the same amounts of calcium and vitamin D as whole milk.

9. A plain baked potato contains no fat, while a typical order of homestyle fries gets about 35 percent of its calories from fat. Piling on the toppings—butter, sour cream, shredded cheese, bacon bits—can shoot the fat content of that baked potato well over the level of fries, though.

10. Sweet and steaming, a lobster tail gets 16 percent of its calories from fat. By comparison, 75 percent of the calories in a grilled filet mignon come from fat. But the drawn butter that accompanies that lobster tail more than makes up for any fat savings. Butter is all fat, 75 percent of which is saturated.

# Staying Connected with Your Partner During Menopause

Midlife is often a time of becoming true to yourself and your needs. If children are in the picture, they are nearly grown or may already have moved out on their own. Careers are well established. Many women find the fourth and fifth decades of their lives to be times of refocusing on their own interests. With all the other changes taking place in her body, especially those involving thought processes and emotions, a woman might well see menopause as a time to come clean about her real feelings. (See Chapters 10, "A Shift from Left Brain to Right Brain," and 11, "Take a Ride on the Wild Side: Mood Swings.")

The result is often a change in sex drive. A woman might no longer be so driven by what others need, including her partner. When she's in bed, what she might really want most to do is sleep. Sex might not be that high on her priority list. Or, she may realize that she has suppressed her sexual desires during the years she spent raising a family and cultivating a career, and is now raring to indulge them.

## Understanding and Expressing Your Needs

What do you want and need? Many women don't really think much about their own needs during their younger decades, when their lives focus on meeting the needs of others. More sex, less sex, variety, predictability—options weren't necessarily considerations earlier in life. If you're not accustomed to talking with your partner about sex, getting started can feel awkward and uncomfortable. But it's the only way to let your partner know what you want. And communication is a two-way process in which you can learn about your partner's desires, too. Satisfaction in a relationship relies on both giving and receiving.

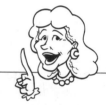

**Wise Woman's Wisdom**

"The process of maturing is an art to be learned, an effort to be sustained. By the age of 50 you have made yourself what you are, and if it is good, it is better than your youth."

—Marya Mannes

## Maintaining Reasonable Expectations

Some women find that while they easily and frequently reached orgasm during sex when they were in their 20s and 30s, by the time they reach age 40 and beyond, orgasm becomes elusive. This is often a cumulative effect resulting from the many changes that take place in your body during the menopause transition. Worrying about it adds to your dissatisfaction and stress. Instead, talk with your partner about your needs. Things change for men during midlife, too. Gradually declining testosterone levels mean that their erections take a little longer to develop, may not always be as firm, and need a longer recovery time to return. Odds are, your partner's needs and desires are changing as well. Extended foreplay leads to enjoyable lovemaking for both of you. Learn to enjoy the journey as much as you enjoy its destination.

# Keeping a Healthy Perspective and Positive Self-Image

In a culture that worships youth, it's sometimes difficult and disappointing to look in the mirror and realize that your youth is behind you. But your prime is in front of you. At last, you have the knowledge and wisdom of experience to guide your choices and actions. You know what you want and what you don't want, and you are less influenced by the opinions of others. Yes, your body is changing. Accept it, and do what you can to keep it healthy and strong. The power of your maturity can take you to new heights, if you let it.

---

### The Least You Need to Know

➤ The physical changes that take place in your body during menopause can affect your sexual desires and responses.

➤ Menopause is a time of change and contemplation during which challenges or problems in relationships sometimes surface.

➤ There are many pleasurable ways to adapt to your body's changes to enjoy an active and loving sex life.

➤ The changes in metabolism that accompany menopause cause your body to need fewer calories. Regular exercise and nutritious eating habits are especially important now.

➤ Men's bodies change during midlife, too. Discussing your feelings and needs can draw you and your partner closer and can deepen your relationship.

---

# Part 4

# HRT or No HRT, That Is the Question

*There's more misinformation and misunderstanding about hormone replacement therapy (HRT) out there than there is knowledge and fact. In large part, this is because no generation before yours had such overwhelming choices. Technology now provides endless options for managing short-term discomforts as well as long-term health risks. And as our technological capabilities grow, we learn more about new ways to use familiar treatments—and about unexpected outcomes, both good and not so good.*

*The next three chapters present a summary of what we know today about the benefits and risks of HRT. This information is by no means definitive, but it provides a good foundation of knowledge to equip you for further explorations of the options most appropriate for you.*

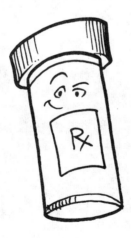

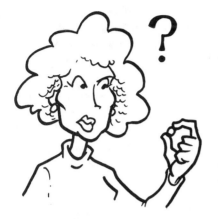

# Chapter 14

# What Is Hormone Replacement Therapy (HRT)?

---

### In This Chapter

➤ The basic kinds of hormone replacement therapy

➤ The benefits and risks of HRT

➤ How HRT affects your risk for heart disease

➤ How HRT affects your risk for cancer

➤ How HRT affects your risk for osteoporosis

---

Among the many medical advances that surfaced in the middle of the twentieth century was the development of a drug called Premarin. Made from purified estrogen compounds extracted from the urine of pregnant horses, this drug miraculously vanquished many of menopause's discomforts. A revolution was born, and within 30 years Premarin was the most commonly prescribed medication in the United States.

Today there are many forms of hormones for replacement therapy. All aim to alleviate the discomforts of menopause and to provide long-term protection against conditions such as osteoporosis without creating additional health concerns such as cancer. How well HRT accomplishes this objective for you depends a lot on your individual situation and your health history.

## OHT, HRT, ERT ... Arrhhh!

If declining hormone levels are the cause of menopause's discomforts, it makes sense to use hormone supplements to restore hormone levels to a point where discomforts disappear. Ah, if only it were that simple! But the human body is an amazingly complex structure, and nothing is quite as easy as it looks. Every woman's body is unique, so there are different approaches for different circumstances. Your menopause signs, any existing health conditions, and your family history of health conditions such as osteoporosis, heart disease, and cancer all are important factors in determining which, if any, form of hormone replacement therapy is for you.

Let's start by sorting through the lingo. Most frequently you'll hear hormone replacement therapy referred to by its acronym, HRT. This has become a broad term encompassing the range of hormone therapies. Estrogen replacement therapy, or ERT, replaces only estrogen. OHT, or ovarian hormone therapy, is sometimes used to refer to hormone replacement therapy that includes estrogen, progesterone, and testosterone—the three ovarian hormones. For our purposes, we'll stick with the term HRT to broadly cover all forms of hormone replacement therapy.

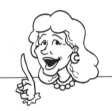

**Wise Woman's Wisdom**

"In youth, a woman gives up her blood to nurture other life. In age, she keeps it to nurture her own wisdom."

—Norwegian saying

## The Benefits of Taking HRT

There are short- and long-term benefits to HRT. In the short term, HRT relieves unpleasant menopause signs such as hot flashes and memory problems. In the long term, HRT prevents or slows osteoporosis and may reduce the risk for heart disease. Recent studies have linked estrogen replacement to protection against Alzheimer's disease and colon cancer.

About three-fourths of women who take HRT do so primarily for short-term relief during the transition through menopause. Less than a third of women continue taking HRT once menopause is complete. Some of them stop because their discomforts are gone. Others pull the plug on HRT out of fear about its long-term risks, which remain uncertain. Despite the uncertainties and sometimes conflicting findings about HRT's long-term effects, many health experts believe that the benefits of HRT outweigh the risks for most women.

Here's a summary of HRT benefits:

➤ HRT provides relief from many of menopause's discomforts, including hot flashes and memory lapses.

➤ HRT lowers blood lipid levels, which may reduce the risk of heart disease and stroke.

➤ HRT improves the ability of your bones to store calcium and make new bone tissue, reducing your risk for osteoporosis by as much as 80 percent.

➤ HRT enhances your brain's chemistry, protecting against memory loss and Alzheimer's syndrome.

➤ HRT lowers your risk for colon cancer.

# The Risks of Taking HRT

Just as there are short- and long-term benefits to HRT, there are long- and short-term risks. Long-term risks generate the greatest concern for most women, particularly because experts don't agree on what those risks are and how significant they should be in making the HRT decision. The risk most women worry about is that of cancer.

In the beginning of HRT, as is typical when medical treatments are new, researchers didn't have enough data to know what effects HRT would have 20, 30, or even 40 years down the road. Early HRT used estrogen alone because this was the hormone that produced relief from menopause's discomforts. For many women, the effects were positive—less chance of heart disease, stronger bones, improved energy, and increased interest in sex. For some women, however, early benefits turned dark in their later years when they developed breast or uterine cancer. Researchers soon linked certain kinds of these cancers to estrogen and then discovered that adding progesterone to HRT helped offset the added risk.

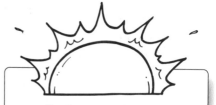

**Embracing Change**

Family history is an important factor in making your HRT decisions. It's helpful to learn as much as possible about the health status of your parents and grandparents on both your mother's and your father's sides. If you don't have access to such information, you and your doctor should carefully consider your personal health history and any clues it might reveal.

The short-term risks of HRT are typically problems that go away when you switch to a different form of HRT or stop taking HRT. Doctors consider these side effects (though if you're experiencing them, they can be more than "side" matters). Bloating (fluid retention), tender breasts, and cramping similar to what you might have had during menstruation affect about 10 percent of women who take HRT. Women whose HRT includes progesterone (which yours should, if you have your uterus) often experience breakthrough bleeding, similar to menstrual periods. Although this goes away in most women, for some women it becomes a problem that ends only when they stop taking HRT.

Here's a summary of HRT risks:

➤ HRT increases your risk for endometrial cancer *only if* you have your uterus and are taking only estrogen.

➤ HRT may increase your risk for certain kinds of breast cancer.

➤ HRT may increase your risk for blood clots, especially in your legs.

➤ HRT that includes progesterone may worsen some menopause discomforts, such as mood swings and depression.

➤ HRT that includes testosterone (androgens) may raise your blood cholesterol levels, cause male-pattern body hair to grow, and deepen your voice.

**151**

# The Kinds of Hormone Replacement Therapy

There are literally dozens of variations for HRT. Most center on three core kinds of hormone replacement: estrogen only, estrogen-progesterone combination, and estrogen or estrogen-progesterone with androgens. It may take some experimentation to find the variation that works best for you, so be patient as well as persistent. Unless you have serious side effects (such as heavy bleeding or significant fluid retention), give an HRT variation several months to prove itself before deciding that it doesn't work for you. Talk with your gynecologist about what to expect and how long to wait for results. But don't hesitate to ask for a change when it becomes clear that your HRT isn't doing what you expected to relieve your menopause discomforts.

## *Estrogen Replacement*

Estrogen is the key player in HRT—and in the beginning of HRT, it was the only player. Estrogen gets credit for all of HRT's benefits: ending hot flashes, strengthening bones, lowering cholesterol, and stabilizing moods. If you no longer have your uterus, your HRT will usually contain only estrogen (see the discussion about progesterone in the next section). Estrogen replacement does not restore ovulation, however. Remember, a key trigger of menopause is that your ovaries stop producing eggs. Nonfunctioning follicles close, and your body reabsorbs any eggs within them. Replenishing your body's estrogen can't bring back what isn't there any more.

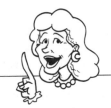

### Wise Woman's Wisdom

"The world is round, and the place which may seem like the end may also be the beginning."

—Ivy Baker Priest

## *Combined Estrogen–Progesterone Replacement*

If you still have your uterus, your HRT should include progesterone as well as estrogen. Progesterone, most commonly in the form of progestin, sustains the endometrium (the interior walls of the uterus). This offsets any potential increased risk of endometrial (uterine) cancer from taking estrogen. Beyond this, progesterone is not given alone as a treatment for the discomforts of menopause (except natural micronized progesterone, especially in the form of a vaginal cream, which doctors sometimes prescribe for hot flashes and vaginal dryness).

Some women whose HRT includes progesterone find that their mood swings and even depression worsen rather than improve. Because progesterone causes the uterus to build up and then shed its lining, adding it to HRT often produces periodlike cyclical bleeding in many women. Although this generally goes away within six months to a year, it can be a frustration for women whose periods had stopped before they started taking HRT. There is also some concern that progesterone reduces the protective ability of estrogen in reducing the risk of heart disease. Because progesterone wasn't routinely added to HRT formulations until the 1970s, there isn't as much long-term data for doctors to fully understand the functions of progesterone in HRT.

Despite the uncertainties that surround the role of progesterone, the evidence is clear that it offsets the potential for increased risk of cancer that's associated with estrogen replacement therapy alone. So, if you have your uterus, the only safe way for you to get the benefits of estrogen replacement is to also take progesterone replacement.

## Androgen Replacement

Some studies suggest that adding a tiny dose of testosterone to HRT helps restore energy and sex drive. So far, however, no study has conclusively demonstrated that this produces consistent benefits. There is concern that adding testosterone to HRT could reduce estrogen's ability to protect against heart disease. Testosterone causes your blood cholesterol level to rise, which contributes to *arteriosclerosis*.

Other risks with androgen replacement include masculinization—male-pattern facial and body hair, a deepening voice, and bulkier muscles. These effects, if they do occur, go away after you stop the androgen replacement. If low sex drive and lack of energy are problems for you that don't go away with regular HRT, discuss the pros and cons of adding testosterone to your HRT on a trial basis.

## If You've Had a Hysterectomy

If you've had a hysterectomy, you don't need progesterone in your HRT. The only role of traditional progesterone replacement is to protect the lining of the uterus. The reason for your hysterectomy might influence your decision on whether to take estrogen replacement therapy, or ERT. Because there is a correlation between estrogen and an increased risk for cancer of the uterus, doctors generally don't recommend estrogen replacement if you've had endometrial or cervical cancer.

**Wise Up**

**Arteriosclerosis** is a condition that occurs when the walls of your arteries become lined with fatty deposits. This causes your arteries to narrow and stiffen, reducing the amount of blood that can flow through them. Severe arteriosclerosis can block blood flow entirely, causing a stroke or a heart attack.

# If Menopause Is So Natural, Why Replace Hormones?

Hormone replacement to offset the signs and consequences of menopause is controversial among women as well as among doctors. A little more than half of American women do choose not to use HRT during or after menopause. They make this decision for a variety of reasons. They might have few menopause-related discomforts. They might not know that HRT is an option, or they might fear the conflicting research findings. They might not have insurance coverage or the resources to pay for HRT. Or, they might decline HRT because they feel that it's unnatural.

After all, nature designed our bodies to function in the way they do, so what right do we have to meddle with the natural order of things? Well, let's take a look at that natural order, which has changed significantly since humankind established its presence on the planet. Consider that just 100 years ago, life expectancy was half of what it is today. Through lifestyle improvements and medical advances, we've altered nature's plan. But nature hasn't kept pace with our alterations. Our bodies still function as they did when 50 was old age, not midlife.

**Wise Up**

**Premenstrual syndrome (PMS)** is a collection of discomforts that precedes a woman's menstrual period. PMS commonly includes cramping, fluid retention, breast tenderness, headaches, irritability, and moodiness. PMS abates within a day or two of the period's start.

It's entirely possible that over the next few centuries, natural changes will occur in our bodies to match our extended life spans, making interventions such as HRT unnecessary. Until that happens, however, sometimes Mother Nature needs a little boost. For many women, HRT can make the menopause transition feel more natural because it restores a sense of balance. Instead of feeling at odds with your suddenly unpredictable body, you again feel perhaps not in control, but at least in synchronization.

## Is HRT as Good as the Real Thing?

The truth is, no one really knows how well HRT matches your body's natural hormonal balances. After all, HRT is an artificial structure imposed on your body from the outside. There are bound to be at least subtle differences in how your body responds. Some of the more obvious signs of your body's struggle to adapt to this new structure show up in the form of side effects such as cyclical or breakthrough bleeding and fluid retention. However, these are often common complaints of women with *premenstrual syndrome* (PMS), which many experts believe *reflects* a naturally occurring imbalance of hormones related to the menstrual cycle.

## Challenges of Replacing Estrogen

It would be wonderful if there were a process for you to extract and store small quantities of the estrogen your body produces during your childbearing years to give back to your body during menopause. Then you would get a precise match. Unfortunately, this kind of storage and retrieval just isn't possible. So, we go for the next best thing—formulations of estrogen that closely mimic the molecular structure of your body's natural estrogen. These formulations are sometimes difficult for your body to absorb, especially when you take them in pill form. You may need to take a high amount of estrogen just to get a low amount into your bloodstream. New methods such as *transdermal patches* are making it easier to match your body's needs.

# HRT and Heart Health

For several decades, doctors have known that there's some kind of relationship between estrogen and heart health. What continues to elude them is the exact nature of this relationship. Heart disease is relatively rare in women before menopause, and it occurs much less frequently than in men of similar age and health background. All other factors being equal, estrogen seems to account for the difference. Although researchers have studied the correlation between estrogen and heart disease for years, they haven't been able to pin down the precise mechanisms involved. This has caused conflicting reports and recommendations, and much confusion among doctors as well as women trying to make decisions about HRT.

**Wise Up**

A **transdermal patch** is a patch that you place on your skin. It contains a drug that is then absorbed through your skin and directly into your bloodstream.

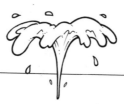

### Wellspring

In the 1990s, the Heart and Estrogen/Progestin Replacement Study (HERS) enrolled nearly 3,000 menopausal women in a research project to zero in on the relationship between estrogen and heart disease. The first findings, published in 1998, reported that HRT had no measurable effect on preventing further heart attacks in women who already had heart disease. Other studies are underway to further explore the relationship between estrogen and heart disease. The most extensive of these is the Women's Health Initiative (WHI), sponsored by the National Institutes of Health. The WHI includes 27,500 women taking HRT and is looking at the long-term effects of HRT on heart attacks, strokes, blood clots, fractures, osteoporosis, and cancer. The WHI is scheduled to conclude in 2005.

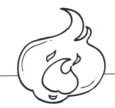

# How Estrogen Affects Cholesterol Levels

Estrogen, the primary hormone in HRT, lowers low-density *lipoproteins* (LDL), or "bad" *cholesterol*, and raises high-density lipoproteins (HDL). High LDL and low HDL levels are known risk factors for heart disease. This effect is not as strong when HRT includes androgen replacement, leading to questions about the relationship between estrogen and testosterone as well as the individual roles these hormones have in how your body handles lipoproteins and cholesterol.

# Your Heart Health: A Self-Quiz

Your risk for heart disease increases as you grow older. Some women are at increased risk for heart disease because of lifestyle factors (they're overweight or obese, they eat a high-fat diet, they don't exercise) or family history. These questions can help you assess your risk for heart disease. Put a check mark beside each statement that is true for you:

1. I participate in aerobic activities (such as swimming, jogging, bicycling, and aerobic dance) for at least an hour three or four days a week.

2. I walk at a moderate to brisk pace for 30 minutes a day, four or five days a week.

3. My weight is appropriate for my height or my BMI (body mass index) is within the normal range.

4. I eat more fruits than pastries and sweets.

5. I eat more grains and vegetables than dairy products and meats.

6. Neither my parents nor my siblings had a heart attack before age 60.

7. My blood pressure is 140/70 or below.

8. My total blood cholesterol level is 200mg/dl or below.

9. I don't have diabetes.

10. I don't smoke.

If you checked seven or more statements, your risk for heart disease is probably normal for your age. If you checked five or fewer statements, you could make some lifestyle changes that would decrease your risk for heart disease. Two risks that you can't influence are family history and diabetes. If these risks exist for you, it's especially important to do all you can to keep your other risks low. And if you didn't check statement 10, your risk for heart disease is much higher than normal. Cigarette smoking is the leading cause of heart disease—and heart disease kills more women each year than all forms of cancer combined. Please quit!

## HRT and Heart Disease

A woman's risk for heart disease increases most dramatically in the first five years following menopause. It then levels out for a decade or two—higher than at any point in a woman's life, but remains lower than the risk for a man of the same age. When you enter your 70s, your risk for heart disease begins to climb again.

Conventional wisdom has held that HRT offers some protective benefits against heart disease, though recent research studies are calling this belief into question. HRT appears to lessen the rate at which your risk for heart disease increases in the second through fifth years after menopause. If you already have risk factors for heart disease (such as family history, diabetes, or cigarette smoking), however, recent studies suggest that HRT may increase your risk for heart attack during the first year after menopause that you take HRT.

Does this mean HRT is bad for your heart? Not necessarily. It means that the decision to take HRT is becoming increasingly individualized. Doctors and women can no longer look at HRT in a general way. What is right for you depends on your unique health picture. You and your doctor must weigh the pros and cons for you personally. Research into the precise ways in which HRT affects your body, in the short term as well as over the long term, continues.

Many variables must combine to establish heart disease, and many of them are within your ability to influence or control. You can knock off a huge chunk of risk,

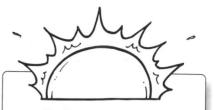

**Embracing Change**

Cigarette smoking increases your risk for a host of health problems that could lower the benefits that you might otherwise receive from HRT. If you smoke, talk with your doctor about resources to help you stop. You're never too old to quit!

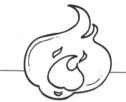

**Hot Flash!**

Beware media reports about research studies. Most excerpt small findings without giving their context. Some studies involve very small numbers of participants and may not apply to women in general. If a media report interests or concerns you, ask your doctor about it or track its source to get the complete picture.

for example, by not smoking—smoking is the leading cause of heart disease in men and women, hormones notwithstanding. Other factors that health experts consider environmental (in contrast to hereditary factors), such as diet and exercise, significantly affect your risk for heart disease. Chapter 27, "Staying Healthy After Menopause: Inner Changes," discusses HRT and heart disease in detail.

# How Estrogen Affects Your Cancer Risks

The cells that cause endometrial cancer and certain forms of breast cancer are hormone-driven—that is, they thrive on the hormones that reach them through your bloodstream. Taking progesterone replacement with your estrogen replacement protects your endometrial cells from the changes that lead to cancer, essentially nullifying any added risk from taking estrogen replacement.

The correlation between estrogen replacement and breast cancer is less clear. For many years, most studies reported little or no increased risk for breast cancer with HRT. But as study methodologies have become more sophisticated, and as the number of women who have taken HRT for 20 to 40 years has increased, the findings are showing some connections. Now researchers suggest that the risk of breast cancer increases by 10 percent for every 10 years that a woman takes HRT. But before you panic, let's put those percentages into perspective. A woman has about a 1 in 12 chance of developing breast cancer if she lives to age 85—about 8 percent. Ten years of HRT could increase this risk to 1 in 11 or so.

The picture is different for women with a family history of breast cancer or who have had breast cancer themselves. Most experts advise against HRT in such situations because there isn't enough information about how HRT influences the risk for developing or advancing cancer. Because estrogen is known to fuel many forms of breast cancer, it makes sense to avoid it unless there are significant risk factors for heart disease.

# Is HRT Good for Your Bones?

One area where HRT shines is in its ability to prevent, or at least significantly slow, osteoporosis. Women who take HRT for a year see their risk for osteoporosis drop by 60 percent. This is significant because by about age 70 or so, without HRT nearly every woman has some degree of osteoporosis. Recent research suggests that the benefits of HRT may last only as long as you continue taking it, presenting strong evidence supporting the need for some level of estrogen replacement that extends beyond menopause.

## *Osteoporosis, Estrogen, and Your Bones*

When you get older, your body becomes less efficient at extracting calcium from the foods you eat. Your body uses calcium for many purposes, among them to contract muscles, clot blood, and transmit nerve signals. If there isn't enough calcium in your bloodstream, your body turns to the "Bank of Bone" and withdraws calcium from your bones. Estrogen halts this process, although scientists aren't entirely sure how. Estrogen also improves the ability of cells to use the calcium that enters your body from what you eat. Estrogen does not seem to help much with the process of rebuilding lost bone tissue, however, so other treatments are necessary once such loss has occurred.

## *Your Osteoporosis Risk: A Self-Quiz*

Every woman's risk for osteoporosis increases with age, as metabolism changes and calcium absorption and depletion become problems. Some women are at increased risk for developing this potentially debilitating medical condition. What is your osteoporosis risk? Put a check mark beside each statement that is true for you:

1. I participate in weight-bearing activities (such as walking, jogging, and weight-resistance training) for at least an hour three or four days a week.

2. I walk whenever possible.

3. My weight is appropriate for my height (or my BMI is within the normal range).

4. I eat or drink three or four servings of low-fat or nonfat dairy products every day.

5. I drink a glass of calcium-fortified milk every morning with breakfast.

6. I eat calcium-fortified cereals and breads.

7. I do not drink cola soft drinks.

8. I take a daily calcium supplement to assure that I get 1,500 milligrams of calcium each day.

9. My mother does not have low bone density, frequent fractures, or osteoporosis.

10. Neither my sisters nor my aunts have low bone density, frequent fractures, or osteoporosis.

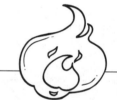

**Hot Flash!**

Are you a "cola-holic"? Cola soft drinks contain high levels of phosphoric acid, which, when it gets into your system, dissolves calcium from your bones. If you must drink soda, select something other than cola or root beer.

If you checked seven or more statements, your osteoporosis risk is probably no greater than average. Weight-bearing exercise and adequate calcium intake are your greatest defenses against bone loss. If you didn't check either statement 9 or statement 10, family history boosts your risk for osteoporosis significantly higher than average.

## *Your Bone Health Without HRT*

For much of their lives, many women can maintain strong, healthy bones with a regimen that includes a nutritious diet that controls weight, calcium supplements to assure a daily calcium intake of 1,500 milligrams, and vigorous weight-bearing exercise. Such an approach is a lifestyle commitment, and it depends on your good health. Because it doesn't take long to undo all your good work, this approach works only if you can give it absolute consistency.

Without a strong lifestyle approach or HRT, your risk for osteoporosis continues to rise as you grow older. It's possible to lose as much as 1 percent of your bone mass a year, which can put you at critical depletion in 10 years. If you already have additional risk factors for osteoporosis—family history or low bone density—your bones without HRT may become frail and fragile before you know it. Although there are medications to help rebuild bone mass, such treatment is not nearly as effective as prevention. Chapter 27 discusses osteoporosis in detail.

---

### The Least You Need to Know

➤ Estrogen replacement stops or slows calcium loss, lowers blood cholesterol levels, and eases many of the discomforts of menopause.

➤ The link between HRT and heart disease is controversial. Discuss your personal risks for heart disease with your doctor when considering HRT.

➤ If you have your uterus, taking estrogen alone increases your risk for certain types of cancer. You should take HRT that combines estrogen and progesterone.

➤ It's important to understand your doctor's position regarding HRT and to seek care from a doctor whose position is a good match with yours.

➤ It often takes several trials of different HRT combinations and methods to find one that works for you.

➤ Media reports about HRT often take study findings out of context, distorting their significance.

---

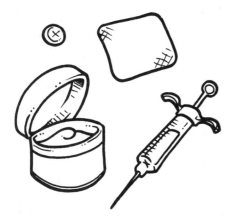

# Chapter 15

# Taking HRT: What's Your Preference?

## In This Chapter

➤ Natural and synthetic products: What's the difference?

➤ The kinds of estrogen, progesterone, and testosterone supplements

➤ Forms and dosages of HRT

➤ Is HRT a lifelong commitment?

➤ Birth control pills as an alternative to HRT

How do you want to take your HRT? There are a number of choices with the products now available. Some preparations are available for different administration methods. Others depend on what strength and type of estrogen, progesterone, or testosterone your doctor wants to prescribe for you. Often it's a matter of personal preference. Some women like the ease of biweekly skin patches, while others prefer daily pills.

There are 50 or more different HRT products on the market, with more likely to debut as they gain FDA approval. This chapter covers the various HRT products in an overview manner. If the HRT your doctor wants to prescribe isn't specifically listed here, don't worry. We just don't have room to list everything, so we've selected the most common products.

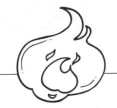

**Hot Flash!**

Don't just stop taking HRT if you decide that you no longer want to go the HRT route. This can put your body into sudden estrogen withdrawal, causing severe hot flashes and other unpleasant experiences. Talk with your doctor about the best way to taper off.

# What Does It Mean to Take HRT?

HRT is a commitment. Although HRT is not difficult to take, it does require you to take the method of HRT that you've chosen in the way it needs to be taken to be effective. If you choose to take cyclical combination estrogen-progesterone pills, for example, you need to take your pills according to the schedule of the cycle. If you choose a transdermal patch instead, you have to be willing to wear it and change it as prescribed. Missed or irregular doses diminish HRT's effectiveness. It can take a few months to know how well your HRT will relieve your menopause discomforts. Many experts feel that it's necessary to take HRT for at least five years to gain any long-term protection from conditions such as osteoporosis, and some believe that women need to take HRT for the rest of their lives to reap its full benefits.

Certainly, you can change your mind about your HRT decision, from the combination, dose, and method that you want to use, to whether to take it at all. Talk with your doctor about changes that you want to make so that you can make them without causing yourself more discomfort.

## Does HRT Reverse Menopause?

Although HRT calms or ends most of the signs of menopause, it doesn't actually halt or reverse menopause itself. The amounts of estrogen (and progesterone, if you're taking combination HRT) are high enough to relieve signs such as hot flashes, but not high enough to restore your body's hormones to their premenopause levels. No amount of estrogen supplementation can give you more eggs, either, so this function of your ovaries does not return. Even with HRT, your follicle-stimulating hormone (FSH) level remains high. Menopause is a transition your body will complete, with or without HRT. HRT's role, in the short term, is to make the transition less traumatic.

## All About Estrogen

Estrogen is the workhorse of HRT. Your body's fluctuating estrogen levels are responsible for all the signs and discomforts of menopause that you may experience, from hot flashes to brain drain. So, HRT's primary goal is to get enough estrogen into your body to subdue these experiences. One challenge with supplemental estrogen is that it's not easy for your body to absorb. Newer formulations attempt to make supplemental estrogen more *bioequivalent* to your body's natural estrogen. Because so many forms of estrogen are available, and because every woman's biochemistry is unique, it can be difficult to choose the one that will work best for you without some trial and error.

When it comes to choosing between synthetic and natural products, most people assume that natural is better. This is not necessarily true, though. Products that are natural (derived from sources found in nature) but not native to the human body could turn out to be more harmful than products that are synthetic (manufactured in a laboratory and bioequivalent to forms found in the human body). So, sometimes synthetic is more natural, as far as your body is concerned!

### Wise Up

A **bioequivalent** substance is one that precisely matches the molecular and chemical structure of a substance found naturally in your body. To your body, it is indistinguishable from the natural substance.

## Synthetic Estrogens

Synthetic estrogens are manufactured in laboratories from chemicals that are similar but not identical to the chemicals in your body that form your body's hormones. Because synthetic estrogens do not exactly match the hormones your body produces, your body works harder to convert them into usable forms. Synthetic preparations often contain stronger concentrations of estrogen to accommodate the waste that occurs during metabolism. Synthetic estrogens are popular because they are less costly and more consistent to manufacture than natural estrogens. Most of the studies that have been done about HRT have involved synthetic estrogens because this is the form of HRT that has been around the longest.

## Natural Estrogens

Natural estrogens are manufactured from plant sources and are chemically identical to the estrogens that occur naturally in your body. Because they are bioequivalent, these preparations are easier for your body to metabolize and use. There are no byproducts that are unfamiliar to your body, so your liver and kidneys handle them with the same ease that they handled the hormones that your body produced during your menstruating years. Micronization is a process that increases the surface area of the product's active hormone ingredients, improving their ability to be absorbed into your system. Think of salt—a single large chunk of salt takes a long time to dissolve in a glass of water. But if you crush the chunk into tiny pieces, the salt dissolves much faster.

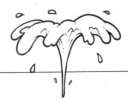

**Wellspring**

Most drugs become available in generic formulations when the original patent on the drug expires. Premarin is a notable exception. Premarin was first approved for use in 1942, when drug manufacturers were not required to isolate each active ingredient and document its effects. The FDA's Center for Drug Evaluation and Research determined in 1997 that it is not possible to identify all of Premarin's active ingredients because it's manufactured from purified extracts from a natural and unquantifiable source. Because approval of generic drugs depends on their bioequivalency to brand-name preparations, the FDA has determined that it cannot grant approval for any generic forms of Premarin.

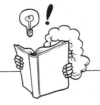

**Wise Up**

A product containing **conjugated estrogens** contains two or more different forms of estrogen in combination. The word *conjugated* means "joined" or "combined" and shares the same linguistic root as the word *yoke*.

## Animal-Based Conjugated Estrogens

The most common form of *conjugated estrogens* is processed and purified from the urine of pregnant mares (female horses). Your liver converts conjugated estrogens into two forms of estrogen for your body to use: estradiol and estrone. Estradiol is the form that does the most to relieve the discomforts of menopause and to provide protection against osteoporosis and heart disease. More than eight million American women take Premarin, the only brand-name product for this formulation that's available in the United States. Although animal-based conjugated estrogens come from a natural source (horses), they are considered nonnative because they don't match the forms of estrogen found in the human body.

## Plant-Based Conjugated Estrogens

Plant-based conjugated estrogens derive their ingredients from plant sources of estrogen, or phytoestrogens. Like animal-based conjugated estrogens, they are considered non-native even though they come from natural sources because they are not forms of estrogen native to the human body. Cenestin is the brand name for the only plant-based conjugated estrogens product currently available in the United States.

## Common Estrogen Products

| Brand Name | Active Ingredients | Source | Method |
|---|---|---|---|
| Cenestin | Conjugated plant estrogens | Synthetic | Oral |
| Climara | Estradiol | Natural | Transdermal |
| Estrace | Micronized estradiol | Synthetic | Oral, vaginal |
| Estraderm | Estradiol | Natural | Transdermal |
| EstraTab | Plant-based estrogens | Natural | Oral |
| FemPatch | Estradiol | Natural | Transdermal |
| Premarin | Conjugated equine estrogens and estrone sulfate | Natural | Oral |
| Tri-Est | Estradiol, estrone, estriol | Natural | Oral |
| VagiFem | Estradiol | Synthetic | Vaginal, tablet |
| Vivelle | Estradiol | Natural | Transdermal |

## *Designer Estrogens*

The newest entries into the estrogen supplement arena are the so-called designer drugs, known to doctors as selective estrogen receptor modulators (SERMs). These high-tech formulations attempt to provide the benefits of estrogen replacement without certain risks. Several of these drugs originally emerged as treatments for breast cancer, and then researchers discovered that they also replaced some of estrogen's functions. Because SERMs are so new, doctors don't know what long-term effects they might have. For this reason, doctors typically prescribe SERMs only for women who need the benefits of estrogen replacement but who have health issues that keep them from taking traditional HRT. Research in this area is ongoing.

## Common SERMs

| Drug | Effects | Risks |
|---|---|---|
| Tamoxifen | Sustains lining of uterus; blocks estrogen's effect on breast tissue; builds bone mass; lowers blood | Current protocols recommend taking this for no more than five years |

*continues*

## Common SERMs (continued)

| Drug | Effects | Risks |
| --- | --- | --- |
| | cholesterol (LDL) | cancer |
| Raloxifene (Evista) | Builds bone mass; blocks estrogen's effect on breast tissue; lowers blood cholesterol (LDL) | Long-term risks are unknown; has no effect on uterine lining |

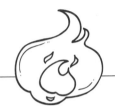

**Hot Flash!**

Mood swings and depression sometimes worsen, or develop if you haven't had them before, when you start taking progesterone. If you notice this with your HRT, contact your doctor. Other HRT methods might not produce this effect.

# All About Progesterone

If you have your uterus, your HRT should include progesterone. There are some exceptions to this, though—for example, if you have a family history of certain forms of breast cancer, or if mood swings are your main reason for taking HRT. If you have your uterus and are taking estrogen-only HRT, be sure that you fully understand your doctor's reason for this choice. There are several ways for you to take progesterone.

## Continuous Progesterone Replacement

Continuous progesterone replacement means that you take progesterone every day, along with your estrogen. The biggest advantage is that you won't experience cyclic bleeding, similar to periods, with this method. You may experience spotty bleeding when you first start taking this form of HRT, but it usually goes away within a few months. The main disadvantage to continuous progesterone replacement is that it can cause unpleasant side effects such as breast tenderness, bloating (fluid retention), and mood swings. If you continue to have these problems, your doctor might suggest that you take your HRT just five days a week, to give your body a break from the progesterone. Several brands of pills are available that contain both hormones, so you take only a single pill. This approach works well for women who have no problems with their HRT, although it is probably not a good first choice in case you need to adjust your doses. You can also use an estrogen patch and take progesterone pills.

## Sequential Progesterone Replacement

With sequential progesterone replacement, you take progesterone only for certain days each month. This emulates your body's natural menstrual cycle, including periodlike bleeding. The bleeding stops over time for many women. The advantage to this approach is that you get progesterone for about the same length of time that your progesterone level would naturally be elevated, reducing the likelihood of unpleasant side effects. If PMS was a problem for you during your menstruating years, you might want to consider HRT that delivers a minimal progesterone dose. The main disadvantage to sequential progesterone replacement is that you must follow a schedule and must remember when to take your progesterone and when not to take it. Many women also find that the cyclic bleeding is something they could do without. If you have side effects with progesterone, your doctor might suggest that you take progesterone less frequently, such as every two or three months.

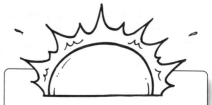

**Embracing Change**

If you're taking sequential progesterone replacement and you have an important event coming, such as a vacation cruise or a long business trip, you can usually skip your progesterone cycle for the month to suppress your monthly bleeding. Check with your doctor first, of course.

## Pulsed (On/Off) Progesterone Replacement

With pulsed, or on/off, progesterone replacement, you take estrogen and progesterone together for three days, and then take estrogen alone for three days. This pattern repeats for as long as you take this form of HRT. The main advantage of pulsed progesterone replacement is that you don't have periodlike bleeding, although you may have spotty or irregular bleeding for a few months after starting HRT. The main disadvantage is that you must keep track of your schedule for taking progesterone, and you must take it consistently. Missing a dose makes it more likely that you'll have breakthrough or spotty bleeding.

### Common Progesterone Products

| Brand Name | Active Ingredients | Form | Method |
| --- | --- | --- | --- |
| Crinone | Natural progesterone | Vaginal gel | Sequential |
| Cycrin | Medroxyprogesterone acetate | Pill | All |
| Nortulate | Norethindrone acetate | Pill | All |
| Prometrium | Natural progesterone | Pill | All |
| Provera | Medroxyprogesterone acetate | Pill | All |

## Common Combination Products

| Brand Name | Active Ingredients | Form | Method |
|---|---|---|---|
| Activella | Estrogen/norethindrone | Pill | Continuous |
| CombiPatch | Estrogen/progesterone | Skin patch | Continuous |
| FemHRT | Estrogen/norethindrone | Pill | Continuous |
| OrthoPrefest | Estrogen/progesterone combination | Pill | Pulse |
| PremPhase | Estrogen/progesterone combination | Pill | Sequential |
| PremPro | Estrogen/progesterone combination | Pill | Continuous |

# What Form and Dose of HRT Is Right for You?

HRT comes in many forms and doses. While this is a blessing in terms of the options it makes available to you, it can also make it more difficult to find the approach that will best meet your needs. There are advantages and disadvantages to each approach. More often than not, you'll need to try several to find one that works for you.

## By Mouth: Pills

The first form of estrogen replacement was a pill, and this remains the most common method of taking HRT. Because your body doesn't very easily absorb estrogen and progesterone through your digestive system, the pills you take contain a much higher amount of hormones than what your body actually uses. Some people have no trouble remembering to take pills according to the prescribed schedule, while other people easily forget or have life circumstances that make a regular schedule difficult (such as a job that involves shifts or extensive travel). Pills are often the least expensive form of HRT.

## By Skin: Transdermal Patches

Transdermal patches deliver HRT through your skin directly into tiny blood vessels. Absorption is usually consistent over a specific period of time. Usually transdermal patches go on your abdomen, and you change them once or twice a week. The primary advantage to transdermal patches is that they can deliver a native form of estrogen, 17 beta estradiol, that is not absorbed well through other methods. Because 17 beta estradiol is bioequivalent to this form of your body's naturally occurring estrogen, there are few side effects.

## *Intravaginally: Vaginal Suppositories and Creams*

Vaginal suppositories and creams deliver HRT through the mucous membranes of the vagina. This form of HRT also helps lubricate the vagina to reduce problems with vaginal atrophy. These forms are most effective when used just before bedtime, so they stay within the vagina until they're fully absorbed. They are less convenient than other forms of HRT.

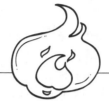

**Hot Flash!**

Progesterone creams are available without prescription. However, most don't contain or deliver enough progesterone to offset estrogen's risk for endometrial cancer (must have a concentration of at least 200 mg/ounce). Using an over-the-counter progesterone cream if you're already taking HRT that includes progesterone could deliver too much progesterone to your body. Over-the-counter progesterone creams are marketed primarily as natural alternatives to relieve PMS and the signs of menopause.

## *By Needle: Intramuscular Injection*

Injected HRT is not a popular choice in HRT, although it offers the advantage that you don't have to worry about taking pills, changing patches, or applying creams. There are several disadvantages. Injectable HRT is estrogen only, and you have to go to the doctor's office once a month to get your shot. It's also possible to have a local reaction at the site of the injection, such as a little redness or itching. The rate at which the injected hormones make their way into your bloodstream is also less predictable than with other forms of HRT. And if you do have an undesirable side effect, it can continue for the duration of the injection's effects.

# Is HRT for Life?

Some experts believe that to receive the maximum benefits of HRT, a woman needs to take it for all of her post-menopausal years—in other words, for the rest of her life. Other experts are concerned that we don't yet know enough about the risks of taking HRT for 30 or 40 or even more years to recommend doing so across the board. There is some evidence that taking HRT for 10 years or longer increases its risks (such as for cancer). There is also evidence that unless you take HRT for at least five years, you don't get much protection against osteoporosis.

Fewer than a third of women who take HRT to ease their transition through menopause continue after menopause is complete. Many women feel that HRT is probably safe in the short term but are reluctant to trust in its long-term uncertainties. How long should *you* take HRT? This is as individual of a determination as the decision to take HRT in the first place, and one that you should discuss with your doctor. If you need the osteoporosis protection, your doctor might suggest a SERM instead of traditional HRT. And it's possible that the next decade will bring new drugs, like SERMs, that offer the benefits of HRT without so many of the potential risks.

## Changing Your Form of HRT

It can take several months for the full effects of HRT to settle in once you start taking it, so it's generally a good idea to give it at least this long before deciding that it doesn't work. It takes time for your body to readjust to its new hormone levels and for those levels to stabilize. This is especially true with side effects such as breakthrough bleeding, which can continue for six months or so before it tapers off. It often takes several trials to find the approach that works best for you. As frustrating as such a process can be, try to be patient. There are dozens of methods and doses for HRT. Generally, there's no need to transition from one form of HRT to another because you're still getting hormone supplements—only the dose or method is changing.

## Stopping HRT

You can decide to stop taking HRT if it's not providing the relief you had hoped it would or because you just don't want to take it any more. Don't just quit taking HRT, though—the sudden withdrawal of hormones will send your body's hormonal equilibrium spiraling out of control. You're likely to experience intensified discomforts until your body readjusts, which can take several months. If you decide to stop HRT because it's not working, talk with your doctor first about trying different forms and doses.

If you choose to stop taking HRT altogether, be sure that you develop and follow a plan to protect your bones and your heart. Eat nutritiously, exercise regularly, and get plenty of calcium (which are all good recommendations even if you continue taking HRT).

# Androgen Therapy

Women also produce androgens, the so-called male hormones. The most abundant of these is testosterone, which, even though it is the most abundant, is still miniscule compared to the level of testosterone in a man's body. With menopause, a woman's testosterone level also drops. Some studies suggest that adding a tiny amount of testosterone replacement to HRT can restore lagging libido (sex drive) and overall energy.

Androgen replacement therapy is more controversial than conventional HRT. Many doctors feel that the lower estrogen and progesterone levels that mark menopause counterbalance the natural decline in a testosterone level. They believe that problems such as low sex drive are related more to other factors such as relationship issues or stress. Other doctors point to the relief of these problems with testosterone supplementation as evidence of its effectiveness.

Testosterone replacement therapy in women is still the subject of research studies. There is much that we don't yet know, especially when it comes to long-term risks and benefits. While testosterone seems to improve estrogen's ability to reduce bone loss, it also increases blood cholesterol levels. Studies still need to assess whether either action is significant. In the short term, testosterone supplementation can produce unwelcome side effects, including male-pattern body hair and a lowered voice. These effects go away after stopping the testosterone supplement.

## Do You Need Testosterone?

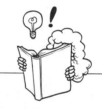

Testosterone supplementation might be a consideration for you if traditional HRT fails to correct problems such as decreased sex drive and lack of energy. Before prescribing a testosterone supplement, your doctor should first do a blood test to measure your levels of testosterone. This test should include both *free testosterone* and *total testosterone,* which then gives a measurement (by calculation) of *bound testosterone.* Because lab tests can't directly measure bound testosterone, it's calculated by subtracting free testosterone from total testosterone. (Chapter 13, "Sexuality, Those 10 Extra Pounds, and Menopause," discusses testosterone levels and how they affect your body.) It's possible for your total testosterone level to be normal and for your free testosterone level to be low, which could account for your symptoms. If your testosterone blood test results are within the range

> **Wise Up**
>
> **Bound testosterone** is attached to proteins in your blood and is inactive (has no effect on body functions). **Free testosterone** is not attached and affects functions such as sex drive. **Total testosterone** is the combination of bound and free testosterone.

of normal values, taking a testosterone supplement is likely to create undesired effects without substantially improving your low energy and sex drive.

## The Testosterone Patch

Administering testosterone through a skin patch seems to provide the best absorption and causes the fewest problems. It's easy and fairly unobtrusive, and it delivers a steady level of testosterone. How often you need to change your patch depends on your dose. You can also take testosterone replacement in pill form or by injection. As with estrogen and progesterone, it's necessary to take a higher dose of testosterone than your body will use when you take pills, because less of the drug is absorbed into your system. Intramuscular injections of testosterone supplement, which are absorbed more slowly than injections directly into a vein but more quickly than a skin patch, can be inconvenient and uncomfortable. With rare exceptions, testosterone replacement accompanies HRT. Several pills are available that deliver a combination of estrogen and testosterone, such as the brand-name product EstraTest.

# Birth Control Pills: An HRT Alternative?

Your doctor may include birth control pills among your options for relieving uncomfortable signs of menopause, particularly if you're in the early stages of your menopause transition (perimenopause). Birth control pills, also called oral contraceptives, contain estrogen and progesterone, the same hormones in HRT, but in much higher concentrations. The formulations usually prescribed to relieve the signs of menopause are low-dose, meaning that they contain the lower doses of estrogen and progesterone than regular birth control pills.

Although birth control pills aren't the same thing as HRT, they can provide the same short-term relief from signs such as hot flashes and mood swings. They have the added benefit of protecting against unplanned pregnancy, which HRT cannot do because of its lower hormone amounts. In fact, taking birth control pills can completely mask your transition through menopause because you'll continue to have monthly periods. You won't ovulate, however, and your body will continue its journey through menopause even though you're not aware of it.

There are some advantages to taking birth control pills. Studies suggest that taking oral contraceptives for 5 to 10 years seems to protect against ovarian, endometrial, and colorectal cancers. This protection extends 10 to 15 years after you stop taking birth control pills. There are also some risks to taking birth control pills, especially if you smoke: You face a significant risk for blood clots and stroke. Women with a history of blood clots or who have heart disease also should not take birth control pills.

Opting for birth control pills delays but doesn't eliminate the need to consider HRT. At some point, you'll need to make a decision about whether to take HRT. Some women switch to HRT when their FSH and estrogen levels indicate that menopause is complete. Others just stop taking birth control pills (although many prefer to taper off rather than abruptly quit, to reduce the potential for discomfort). It doesn't seem to cause any problems to continue taking birth control pills for up to a year or so beyond menopause, although there aren't any studies of longer use. Most doctors suggest that women who want to continue hormone supplementation switch to HRT to reduce the risks of long-term hormone use.

### The Least You Need to Know

➤ It often takes several trials of HRT combinations, methods, and products to find the one that works for you.

➤ There is no single "right" way to take HRT. What's right is what works for you.

➤ The forms of HRT that are easiest for your body to use are those that are bio-equivalent to the hormones that your body produces naturally.

➤ Birth control pills can relieve the discomforts of menopause, but they are not the same as HRT.

173

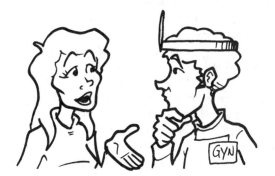

# Making Your Own Decision About HRT

Nearly everyone has an opinion about HRT. Doctors view it from the perspective of health benefits and risks. Women consider the balance of benefits and risks as well as the balance between relief and nuisance. Some women (and doctors) believe the transition through menopause should be natural and without interference from medical technology. Others welcome any assistance that eases the transition's discomforts and challenges. You might begin to feel that everyone else "knows" what's best for you.

Although it's important to learn as much as you can about HRT, in the end the only opinion—and decision—that matters is yours. Each woman has unique circumstances, health variables, and beliefs that shape her HRT decision. You must assess yours and consider all the options that are appropriate for you so that you can make an informed decision. And remember: No decision is carved in stone. You can always change your mind.

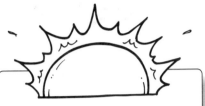

## An Individual Matter

At first glance, your menopause experience might appear just like your sister's or your neighbor's or your co-worker's. When you look a little deeper, however, you'll see subtle and sometimes substantial differences. Perhaps your sister doesn't know what a breast lump feels like, while you've had several breast biopsies that, although the results were benign, have created concern for you and your doctor about breast cancer. Maybe your neighbor's grandmother has had numerous fractures, while the women in your family tree have had high blood pressure (a form of heart disease). Hot flashes that draw attention to your co-worker in staff meetings might be her primary concern, while mood swings could be wreaking havoc in your life. Although HRT might be an appropriate choice for all of you, you all have different needs and risks.

**Embracing Change**

Even though your menopause and HRT experiences will be unique to you, it's often helpful to talk with friends about their experiences. This gives you a broader sense of the diverse scope of the menopause journey, as well as the ways to shape it.

## *What's Right for Someone Else ...*

We like to think of modern medicine as precise and definitive. Take a certain pill, see a certain response. And indeed, that's how it works with many treatments. For the most part, if you take an antibiotic for an infection, the drug will kill the bacteria and the infection will go away. Take an antihistamine, and your allergies subside. Chew a couple antacid tablets, and your stomach settles down. When these results don't occur, you know there's a different problem.

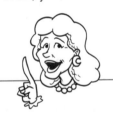

**Wise Woman's Wisdom**

"It's never too late—in fiction or in life—to revise."

—Nancy Thayer

HRT is neither precise nor definitive. It may cut your hot flashes in half, end them altogether, or increase them. There isn't really a problem to blame—your body just has different needs that you haven't yet identified. But you don't know what you'll get until you try. Remember the childhood carnival game of fishing, where you cast your line (a string, tied to a stick, with a clothespin on the end) over a curtain? You never knew what you'd get until you pulled it back. In theory, every item was a wonderful surprise. But sometimes you were thrilled (a yo-yo), and sometimes you were disappointed (a whistle that your mom would take away as soon as you got home).

Now, if you were enterprising, you'd initiate trade negotiations as soon as you saw the same look of disappointment on someone else's face. Then you'd both get what you wanted, and you'd both be happy—even if you all you traded was a red yo-yo for a blue one.

HRT is considerably more complicated than fishing for yo-yos and whistles, of course. But the concept is much the same. You won't know what the results will be for you until you start taking it. Your HRT experience will not be the same as your sister's or your friend's or your neighbor's. What works for them may or may not have the same results for you. Your HRT experience will be uniquely yours, even if you take the same medications as someone you know. This makes it especially important to pay attention to how your body responds to HRT and to contact your gynecologist if those responses are different than you expected.

## Can We Talk? Having a Heart-to-Heart with Your GYN

Your gynecologist is the place to start in determining whether HRT is for you. Your quest should begin with a complete gynecological examination, including a Pap test and a breast exam. Your gynecologist also should collect a comprehensive health history from you—what medical problems you've had, what medical problems your parents and siblings have had, and any current medical concerns.

Then it's your turn to ask the questions. Here are some to get you started:

➤ What HRT does your gynecologist recommend for you, and why?

➤ Does your gynecologist recommend HRT regardless of your menopause experience (even if the signs of menopause are few)?

➤ Is this a general recommendation that your gynecologist starts with for all women who take HRT, or is the recommendation based on your particular situation and needs?

➤ What does your gynecologist expect HRT to accomplish for you?

➤ When should you expect to see results from your HRT?

➤ How long does your gynecologist suggest that you take HRT?

➤ How will your gynecologist monitor your HRT to determine whether it's helping you?

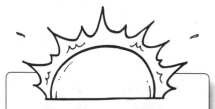

**Embracing Change**

Go to your doctor's appointment well armed with general knowledge about HRT so that he or she can focus on answering questions that are specific to your needs and circumstances. This helps you make the most of your time with your doctor to address your specific concerns.

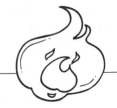

**Hot Flash!**

Although many of the decisions about HRT are ones that you can make based on your personal philosophy and preferences, some are determined by your health history. If your doctor nixes one of your choices, ask for an explanation, but remain open to other options.

It helps to write down your questions before your appointment so that you don't leave any out. You will probably have specific questions that relate to your health (medical conditions or medications that you take already) and family history. Often other questions will occur to you in the course of your discussion. If your gynecologist doesn't have enough time to answer all your questions, schedule another appointment just for the purpose of finishing your discussion. Most gynecologists schedule a longer than usual appointment time for initial HRT evaluations, to accommodate questions and conversation.

Some doctors have strong feelings about HRT, either supporting or rejecting the approach. Most who do will let you know where they stand because they feel so strongly. Some doctors feel that they know what's best for you because they're the experts. Other doctors feel that they should present you with all your options and then let you decide what to do. The majority of doctors are somewhere in between, providing their perspectives based on their experiences, yet willing to collaborate with you to select the HRT option (if any) that best fits your circumstances and meets your needs. As knowledgeable as doctors are, it's always to your advantage to know as much as possible about the options available to you (especially risks and benefits) and to participate in making decisions that affect your health.

# Weighing the Benefits and Risks of HRT

The HRT decision would be much easier to make if the benefits and risks were clear and consistent. Unfortunately, they're not. Even research studies produce conflicting results. Add your personal health history and circumstances to the mix, and sorting through the benefits and risks becomes a monumental challenge. Most women who are considering HRT focus on its ability to relieve the unpleasant physical experiences of menopause. But it's important to remember that there are two components to HRT: short-term relief and long-term benefits. Your decision about HRT must balance both.

## *Characterizing Your Menopause Experience*

For many women, the menopause passage is relatively calm. There might be a few hot flashes here and there, and a mood swing or two. But for the most part, the only noticeable sign is irregular or absent periods. If you are such a woman, you might question whether you even need HRT. Perhaps you don't. About 60 percent of American women go through menopause without HRT, and HRT is significantly less common in many other countries (although natural alternatives such as herbal reme- dies and phytoestrogens are more common). For you, the answer probably depends more on other factors, such as family history.

Most women who are considering HRT have menopause signs that are creating problems in their lives. Hot flashes, mood swings, heavy periods, tiredness, sleep dis- turbances, and depression are among the difficulties that lead women to their gyne- cologists in search of relief. If you are such a woman, the odds are good that taking HRT for three to five years will carry you more comfortably through the remainder of your menopause passage.

## Looking at Your Risk Factors

Family history often takes center stage when con- sidering risk factors, both supporting and opposing HRT. If your grandmother had weak bones and your mother has low bone density, you're at high risk for osteoporosis. Even if your only exposure to hot flashes is what you read and hear other women discuss, you might want to consider HRT for its ability to prevent or reduce osteoporosis. However, if your mother and two of your sisters have had breast cancer, you'll want to carefully weigh HRT's potential benefits against its potential to further increase your risk of getting breast can- cer.

## What HRT Can and Cannot Do for You

HRT can ease the discomforts of your menopause transition, but it can't hold up or turn back the hands of time. Nor can HRT guarantee that you

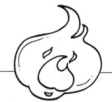

**Hot Flash!**

There is sometimes confusion about what "natural" treatments for HRT include. From a medical perspective, natural treatments are prescribed forms of HRT that are derived from natural (plant and animal) sources. Botanical remedies (such as those we dis- cuss in Chapter 19, "Soy, Herbs, and Other Botanicals: Nature's Menopause Miracles") are con- sidered natural alternatives.

won't have osteoporosis, heart disease, or other health problems related to the changes that your body experiences due to its decreased estrogen and progesterone levels (although it can reduce your risks of developing them). And while HRT restores a higher level of hormones in your body that improves a number of functions, it cannot restore your fertility. Uncertainties about the long-term effects of HRT—both benefits and risks—do remain. Nonetheless, many health experts believe that for most women, the balance clearly tips toward the benefits.

# What HRT Option Is Best for *You?*
# A Self-Assessment

Deciding what kind of HRT is for you is often a process of trial and error. Many doctors have a standard protocol that they follow for women who fit certain general categories—those with uteruses and those without, for example, which divides them into estrogen-only and estrogen/progesterone combination camps. Additional questions further whittle down the options until a few promising choices remain.

You can get a head start on this process by answering some questions before you meet with your doctor. You might photocopy these questions and your responses, and take this list with you to your doctor's appointment. There are no right or wrong answers; the point is to help you identify preliminary concerns and preferences that will shape your HRT decision.

*Your Health Background*

1. Have you had a hysterectomy?
2. Do you have, or have you ever been treated for, any kind of cancer?
3. If the answer to no. 2 is "yes," do you (or did/you) have breast cancer, endometrial cancer, or cervical cancer?
4. Did your mother or sisters have breast, endometrial, or cervical cancer?
5. Do you smoke cigarettes?
6. Do you have high blood pressure or cardiovascular disease?
7. Are you Caucasian?
8. Do you have a slight build?
9. Did you have moderate to severe PMS during your menstruating years?
10. Do you take any regular medications?
11. Did the self-test "Your Heart Health: A Self-Quiz" in Chapter 14, "What Is Hormone Replacement Therapy (HRT)?" identify you as having a higher-than-average risk for heart disease?
12. Did the self-test "Your Osteoporosis Risk: A Self-Quiz" in Chapter 14 identify you as having a higher-than-average risk for osteoporosis?

*Your Menopause Experience*

13. Are you having hot flashes?
14. Are you having mood swings, or are you frequently irritable?
15. Do you feel fatigued and sluggish?
16. Are your periods irregular, unusually light, or unusually heavy?

17. Have your periods stopped altogether?

18. Do you have migraine headaches that you didn't have before your menopause transition began?

19. Do you feel bloated, or are you retaining fluid?

20. Do you have trouble remembering or concentrating on mental tasks?

21. Do you have vaginal dryness or itching?

22. How strong is your interest in sex?

23. Do you have discomfort or pain during sex?

24. Do you feel down, blue, or depressed more often than not?

25. Do you believe that the signs of menopause are inevitable discomforts, or do you believe that you have the right and the ability to shape your menopause transition?

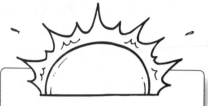

**Embracing Change**

Lifestyle is more important for overall health and well-being than your decision on whether to use HRT. Even with HRT, taking part in regular aerobic and weight-bearing exercise, eating a nutritious diet, using relaxation techniques to relieve stress, and taking time for yourself are all integral to your healthy present, as well as future.

*Your Preferences*

26. Do you have trouble remembering to take medications on a schedule?

27. Does it bother you to think that your regular monthly bleeding might continue for a few more years?

28. Do you have problems taking pills?

29. Does it bother you to think of wearing a patch on your skin?

30. How long do you envision yourself taking HRT?

# Giving Yourself What You Need

This isn't your mother's menopause, a concept we'll come back to in later chapters. The options that you can choose from to make your menopause transition a pleasant passage to the next stage of your life weren't even dreams when your mother and grandmothers before you completed their journeys. Modern medicine may not be able to cure the common cold (yet!), but it can put the chill on hot flashes, steady the pendulum of mood swings, and keep the calcium in your bones. You are among the first of what will be many generations who can not only live to a ripe old age, but who also remain healthy enough to enjoy it.

## High-Tech Medicine for the All-Natural Lifestyle

For some women who strive to live as naturally as possible, the HRT decision can pose a dilemma. How do you remain true to your life philosophy and still meet your body's needs? Intervention isn't necessarily unnatural. Sometimes you need to give your body a boost. Many women use HRT just to get them through the transition phase of menopause. While doctors don't know whether this gives as much long-term protection against conditions such as osteoporosis, it does ease the short-term discomforts.

As you know from the previous chapter, there are now forms of estrogen and progesterone replacement that are derived from natural sources that are chemically identical to human hormones (bioequivalent). These minimize the intrusive nature of HRT and reduce common side effects. And if HRT seems unacceptably unnatural to you under any circumstances, you might be able to bolster your body's hormone needs through natural sources. The chapters in Part 5, "Menopause Treatment *Au Naturel,*" discuss non-HRT approaches.

## Perfecting Your Menopause Balance

Menopause is a time of shifting from a balance of hormones and body activities supporting reproduction to a new balance focused on nonreproductive functions. The challenge is to maintain a sense of balance amidst the shifting, to position yourself on the pivot point of this seesaw of transition in your life. You won't always be able to control your passage, of course. But with knowledge and understanding about the process of menopause and the options available to assist your body on its journey through it, you can smooth your way.

---

### The Least You Need to Know

➤ Your health history helps determine which HRT options are appropriate for you.

➤ Take a copy of your HRT self-assessment with you to your doctor's appointment to help you more efficiently assess your options and make HRT decisions.

➤ Your lifestyle is more important overall than whether you choose to take HRT.

➤ The decision to take HRT is a commitment on your part to follow the HRT dosage schedule. If you don't, HRT will not provide the benefits you expect.

➤ You can always change your mind about HRT.

---

# Part 5
# Menopause Treatment
# *Au Naturel*

*Long before there was HRT, there was Mother Nature to provide an abundance of remedies and tonics for smoothing the bumps along the menopause path. Many of these therapies remain available today, and they are attracting renewed interest among women now embarking on their midlife transitions. Some, like soy, seem near-miracles that erase menopause discomforts. Others are of dubious value beyond the placebo effect. And a few are downright dangerous.*

*The next five chapters take you through the gardens of purported relief, helping you separate the blossoms from the weeds.*

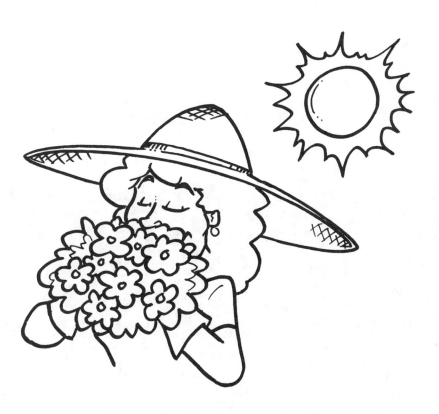

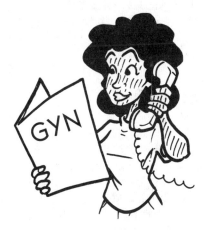

# Taking the Integrative Approach to Menopause

Women have traveled the transforming path of menopause since, well, the beginning of human existence. Across time and cultures, they've passed on various remedies to make the transition easier and more pleasant. Doctors had little, if any, involvement. Menopause was a woman's matter, not a concern for learned men consumed by weightier issues such as how blood traveled through the body and whether the head or the heart was the seat of the soul.

Women made do, as women have always done, with solutions that they found surrounding them in nature. And they made do quite well, given the abundant resources that flourished in the fields and forests. Roots, seeds, stems, and leaves became teas, salves, powders, and other medicinals that soothed not only the discomforts of menopause, but also the symptoms of dozens of ailments, from headaches to bunions.

Now, following a century of amazing medical discoveries that have left few mysteries of the human body unsolved, many women (and often their doctors) are wondering if it's possible to combine the new knowledge of science with the wisdom of ages.

# What Is Integrative Medicine?

*Integrative medicine* attempts to achieve a blend and balance of the various approaches to managing menopause. It views the body as a holistic entity in which the physical, emotional, and spiritual continually interact. It strives to bring the best of all worlds together in ways that are both focused and broad-based, encompassing the full spectrum of the menopause experience. In many respects, integrative medicine is a uniquely Western concept because the medical practices of most other cultures inherently incorporate a broad base of prevention, diagnosis, and treatment methods.

## *The Western Standard: Allopathic Medicine*

The medicine most familiar to Westerners is called *allopathic medicine*. This is the venue of M.D.s and hospitals, diagnostic tests and medical technology, prescription drugs and surgery. Allopathic medicine tends to focus on diagnosing and treating disease conditions through interventions more than on preventing health problems through lifestyle choices. This is changing as we learn more about the relationships among health, disease, and lifestyle. The shift is most apparent in conditions such as heart disease, where there are clear connections to lifestyle practices such as eating and exercising. Although allopathic medicine dominates healthcare in the United States, it's a relative newcomer that didn't really come into its own until the middle of the 1900s.

**Wise Up**

**Integrative medicine** seeks to blend and balance various methods to provide a holistic, or unified, approach to wellness as well as treatment. **Allopathic medicine** is conventional Western medicine practiced by M.D.s (medical doctors) and, often in the United States, by D.O.s (doctors of osteopathy).

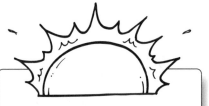

**Embracing Change**

The licensing requirements of American mental healthcare professionals differ among states. Your doctor, medical center, or local hospital can direct you to those in your community who are qualified to help with your particular concerns. It's important to verify the provider's qualifications before entering into any treatment.

Conventional allopathic approaches to the emotional dimensions of transitional life and health experiences such as menopause direct people to counselors, psychotherapists, psychologists, and psychiatrists (M.D.s who specialize in treating mental illnesses). These mental healthcare professionals help people work through the emotional and relationship challenges and issues that confront and concern them.

# Natural Traditions in Healing and Healthcare

Other forms of medicine are based on natural traditions, many of which have been passed through cultures and centuries. Among the most familiar are these:

➤ **Ayurveda,** the traditional medicine of India, has been practiced for more than 5,000 years. Ayurveda bases diagnosis and treatment on three doshas, or types of bodies and personalities. Ayurvedic medicine emphasizes the whole person—physical, emotional, spiritual, and intellectual—rather than processes of wellness or disease. An Ayurvedic physician typically studies for five years at an Ayurvedic medical school and then serves two years in a program similar to the American internship and residency.

➤ **Homeopathy** uses tiny amounts of natural substances to stimulate the body's own healing mechanisms. Homeopathy came into existence in the early 1800s and reached the peak of its popularity in the United States in the late 1800s and early 1900s, after which it gave way to allopathic medicine. This form of medicine remains popular in European countries as well as Russia, India, and Mexico.

➤ **Naturopathy** uses remedies found in nature, such as plants and herbs. In modern practice often incorporates elements of homeopathy, TCM (see the last point in this list), and other forms of complementary medicine. Practitioners who complete their education and training through a school of naturopathic medicine can be licensed as naturopathic doctors, or NDs.

➤ **Osteopathy** views the body as a unified structure, with the musculoskeletal system as its core. Practitioners complete a comprehensive program through a school of osteopathic medicine and can be licensed as doctors of osteopathy, or D.O.s. In the United States, many D.O.s practice allopathic medicine.

➤ **Traditional Chinese medicine (TCM),** another ancient form of medicine, typically incorporates acupuncture and herbal remedies. Practitioners may study for many years in an apprenticeship role before becoming fully qualified to diagnose and treat.

These methods incorporate a spectrum of therapies ranging from acupuncture to vitamins. Many remedies that these traditional approaches use are based in natural substances, such as preparations made from plants and herbs. Others, such as acupuncture, have been known to civilizations since before recorded history. Methods for inducing relaxation are integral components of many natural traditions, although

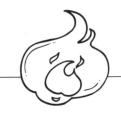

### Hot Flash!

*Always* tell your doctor about any herbal, botanical, and other remedies you're using, whether or not you take HRT. Some preparations can interact with medicines and other treatments, creating unpredictable results. In most situations, it's possible to find a healthy balance as long as you and your doctor are working as partners for your best health.

often are not viewed as separate from methods that target a person's physical needs. These include meditation, guided imagery, hypnosis, yoga, healing touch, therapeutic massage, energy medicine, and martial arts such as tai chi. Such methods emphasize the unity of body, mind, and spirit to achieve health that encompasses the whole being.

## Blending Allopathic and Natural Traditions

Many women and a growing number of doctors believe that no single approach works best in all situations. Some women have health issues that make HRT a necessity, while others may find that HRT creates further problems for them. Most women will experience the menopause that they want to experience when they can select from among the many options that exist along the entire spectrum of healthcare philosophies and practices. And they're finding that one choice doesn't preclude others. You *can* take HRT—in any of its many formulations—and also seek relief from traditional remedies.

## Why Take an Integrative Approach to Menopause?

What Western cultures consider alternative medicine is the convention in many other cultures. More American women take HRT than women in any other country. In European countries such as Germany, there are pharmacological standards for herbal and botanical preparations similar to those that exist in the United States for prescription and over-the-counter drugs. Remedies such as dong quai and ginseng are commonplace (see Chapters 18, "Turning to Nature for Hormone Support," and 19, "Soy, Herbs, and Other Botanicals: Nature's Menopause Miracles").

## The Revolution in Mind-Body Healthcare

The decade of the 1960s was a time of revolution on many fronts. The discovery of the birth control pill spawned what has since become known as the sexual revolution. The war in Vietnam exposed a generation of young Americans to Eastern culture and practices. Television made the world suddenly smaller, beaming other lifestyles into Western living rooms. And interest in more integrative approaches to medical care and health began to grow. Methods that had once seemed exotic or far-fetched were now the subjects of sophisticated, controlled, scientific experiments. *Biofeedback*—a therapy that in its beginning appeared to be part parlor game, part sci-fi—emerged as a legitimate method for reducing the severity of, and even preventing, chronic pain problems such as headaches.

Scientific research in the final decades of the twentieth century produced revolutionary discoveries about the interactions between body and mind. Researchers isolated chemical messengers called *neuropeptides* that affect feelings such as happiness and sadness, appearing to be the biochemical basis for emotions. Scientists also identified other chemical substances called *endorphins* that relieve pain, as well as the neurotransmitters involved in disorders such as Alzheimer's disease that affect cognitive and memory functions, our ability to think and remember. (See Chapter 10, "A Shift from Left Brain to Right Brain.")

This combination of research and access to the traditions of other cultures spurred renewed interest in remedies and treatments beyond the realm of modern allopathic medicine. What began as a movement toward alternative therapies has since evolved into a recognition that these approaches—allopathic medicine included—can coexist in a complementary or integrative manner to provide the best of all worlds when it comes to meeting individual healthcare needs.

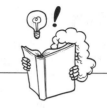

### Wise Up

**Biofeedback** is a learned method of consciously altering physical functions that typically take place without conscious effort. **Neuropeptides** are chemical structures called amino acids that convey messages between the brain and the body. **Endorphins** are morphinelike chemicals the brain naturally produces to relieve pain.

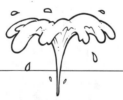

### Wellspring

One of the most widely recognized and extensively documented successes in integrative medicine is the work of American physician Dean Ornish, who has developed a regimen to treat—and even reverse—heart disease. The Ornish program incorporates allopathic diagnosis and treatment with a blend of conventional and complementary therapies, including psychotherapy, meditation, regular exercise, and a low-fat, vegetarian diet. For most people who enter the program, the regimen reflects a complete lifestyle change. In return, they see significant health improvements that often include a stop in the progress of their heart disease or even a return to heart health.

# Getting Integrative Care for Menopause

The concept of integrative care is working its way through the channels of allopathic medicine in many areas of healthcare, as we're all—doctors and women—learning more about the relationship between lifestyle and wellness. A growing number of medical doctors embrace a holistic approach to health and wellness, seeing in it a process for empowering women to manage their own health. Others don't take this approach. If you do, it's important to establish a relationship with a physician who shares your perspectives. This allows you to be open about complementary therapies that you want to try, and allows your doctor to be open about conventional treatments that he or she feels are appropriate for your circumstances.

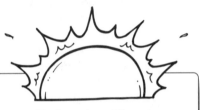

**Embracing Change**

Many metropolitan areas feature holistic health clinics that offer both allopathic and complementary care. If you live in a less urban community, it might be more difficult for you to find healthcare providers who are both willing to and capable of offering integrative healthcare services. It's a good idea to become knowledgeable about the methods and treatments that interest you.

## Start with Your GYN

Although all gynecologists pass the same standardized tests, they are certainly not alike in the way they think about healthcare. Many, but not all, support an integrative approach for lifestyle transitions such as menopause. That's okay. Different women have different preferences and needs, and not everyone wants to integrate a variety of methods into managing her menopause. (That's okay, too.) What matters to you is finding a gynecologist (known more familiarly as a GYN) who thinks the same way you do. If you've been seeing the same GYN for your women's healthcare needs for a number of years, you've probably made this connection already. If not, this is the time to find it.

Most GYNs are willing to schedule informational or interview appointments to give the two of you a chance to compare notes (and most insurance plans cover these visits just as they would cover any other doctor visits, although you should check with yours to be sure). Don't let it make you feel uncomfortable to "interview" your doctor; the two of you are going to be partners in making some of the most important decisions of your life. Are you interested in exploring complementary or natural remedies for your menopause discomforts? Do you think you should take HRT? A combination? Let the GYN know how you feel and what questions you have. Listen to the answers you get, and ask how the GYN feels about the health matters that are important to you.

Remember, too, that the choice you make today isn't one that binds you forever. If you find that you and your GYN don't see eye to eye after all, make a change. The goal is to establish a partnership that respects your health wishes.

## Other Healthcare Professionals Who Can Help

Numerous other healthcare professionals—both allopathic and complementary—can help make your journey through menopause a pleasant one. You might benefit from the recommendations of a nutritionist, who can help you develop a dietary plan that incorporates foods high in isoflavones and other substances to ease the discomforts of menopause and improve your body's ability to maintain good health. A physical therapist or exercise physiologist can help you design a fitness plan to tone and strengthen your muscles and bones. An herbalist can customize a regimen of botanical remedies. Other professionals who can offer assistance include acupuncturists, massage therapists, naturopathic physicians, hypnotists, and psychotherapists. When seeking allied healthcare services such as these, look for professionals with both training and experience in working with women who are going through menopause.

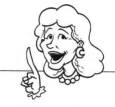

**Wise Woman's Wisdom**

"We grow neither better nor worse as we get old, but more like ourselves."

—May Lamberton Becker

## What About Psychologists?

As a time of life transition, menopause can surface a range of concerns and issues that you've buried, avoided, or not had to deal with before. This is a time when you might be questioning where you've come in your life and where you're going. Many women enter menopause with a sense of satisfaction about the past and look forward to the future. Some women are less certain about one, the other, or both. A qualified mental health professional, such as a psychotherapist or a psychologist, can help you sort through your concerns and help you work through depression or other distressing emotions. A new specialty area is energy psychology, in which psychologists are trained in integrative approaches.

## Building Your Menopause Care Team

Many women who choose an integrative approach to managing their menopause experiences use their gynecologists as their core practitioners. Other practitioners—herbalists, naturopathic physicians, acupuncturists, nutritionists, psychotherapists, and psychologists, to name a few—fill out the circle. Some women choose a complementary practitioner, such as an herbalist or a naturopathic physician, to act as their center of gravity for menopause-related needs. Which do you need on your menopause care team? It depends on your personal circumstances, beliefs, and needs. Your team may change as you make your way through your menopause transition and as your circumstances change.

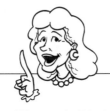

# When Insurance Will and Won't Pay

Many health plans provide at least limited coverage for what they define as alternative or complementary therapies. Some states mandate a certain level of coverage, requiring insurers to pay for a variety of unconventional healthcare services for people enrolled in their insurance plans. The services most likely to be covered include acupuncture and naturopathic medicine. Those least likely to be covered are herbal remedies and vitamin therapies, especially for products available without a physician's prescription.

Insurance companies are likely to view with skepticism treatments for which there are few or no scientific studies confirming their merits, and they often refuse coverage on the basis that such treatments are experimental. This is the case with allopathic as well as complementary therapies, although often this occurs more frequently with complementary approaches because there are fewer studies of them.

Some insurance plans will cover complementary therapies when your allopathic physician gives you a formal referral for them. In such situations, your doctor provides a medical reason for the services. And, in some circumstances, you can challenge your insurance company's refusal to pay for complementary care, although this varies among policies and states. Some policies pay only for services explicitly listed, while others pay for those that aren't explicitly excluded. Confused? You're not alone! It's worthwhile to check the fine print of your health plan.

Having your health insurance pay for your healthcare choices certainly makes your decisions easier. Rather than focusing on cost, you can look at what might help your particular discomforts and how it fits with your beliefs and desires about menopause and healthcare. Few people have all their healthcare decisions covered by their health insurance plans, however. You often have to make choices that involve paying directly for care and therapies. This is yet another reason to understand the potential benefits and risks of the therapies you want to use.

Some medical centers have started offering complementary healthcare services along with traditional therapies. In such an environment, you might receive healing touch as part of presurgical counseling, for example, or see an herbalist as well as a nutritionist and a pharmacist. If these services interest you but aren't available where you regularly receive care, tell your doctor and your insurance company. If integrative care becomes an important issue for enough people, its availability will increase.

# Menopause Management: It's Your Life, and You're in Charge!

This is your life, and this is your menopause. It's your right (and your responsibility) to shape the experience that you want to have. Of course, you can't control every aspect of your menopause transition, but you can direct its general course. Not choosing is nonetheless a choice that often leaves decisions in the hands of others who, although they mean well, don't know you and your needs as well as you do. When you think about it, the opportunities you have right now are pretty astounding. There are few other passages in your life over which you can have so much influence. Take charge while you can!

---

### The Least You Need to Know

➤ What Western cultures view as alternative healthcare is the standard in many other cultures.

➤ Conventional allopathic medicine is beginning to understand and value the role of lifestyle in maintaining health.

➤ Many, although not all, gynecologists welcome the holistic approach of integrative healthcare.

➤ A number of states require insurance companies to include coverage for complementary therapies for people enrolled in their plans.

➤ With all the options available to you, you can shape the menopause experience that you want to have.

➤ Not every therapy or treatment, whether allopathic or complementary, is for every woman. It's important to make choices that meet your healthcare needs and fit with your interests and lifestyle.

---

193

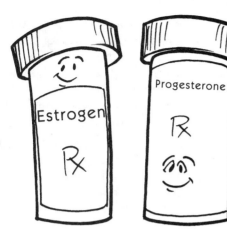

# Turning to Nature for Hormone Support

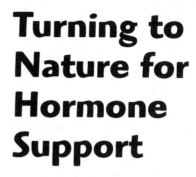

Many women prefer to use natural hormone support to supplement or replace conventional HRT. You might be confused about the conflicting research findings about HRT, or you might have a health history that rules out HRT as an option for you. Or perhaps you just believe that natural is better.

Natural hormone support certainly has its advantages, not the least of which is your ability to pick and choose products that target your unique menopause discomforts. Herbal remedies and botanical preparations feature less concentrated amounts of hormones, making it less likely that you'll experience unpleasant side effects from taking them. This could mean that you won't get the relief you're seeking, however. It might take the same kind of trial and error that HRT often requires to find the combination of natural hormone support that works for you.

# When Are Hormones Natural?

It seems that this would be an easy question to answer. But the answer is not so clear-cut: It depends. From a medical perspective, natural hormones come from sources found in nature (plants) and may or may not be chemically identical to the hormones your body makes. When they are chemically identical to your body's hormones, they're considered native. For example, the HRT product Estrace is synthetic (does not come from a source found in nature) but is native. Premarin is natural but is non-native.

In a broader context, many people draw the line on what's natural between therapies that require a doctor's prescription and remedies that don't. Chapter 15, "Taking HRT: What's Your Preference?" discusses the medical perspective on natural and synthetic hormones. In this chapter, we'll take the broader perspective and look at the range of natural hormone support therapies and menopause remedies that are available for self-management.

## The Difference Between HRT and Natural Hormone Support

HRT is a medical treatment that requires a doctor's oversight. Hormone replacement medications are powerful drugs that are available only from a pharmacy with a doctor's prescription. Before being made available for general use, these drugs undergo extensive testing to determine their effectiveness and to identify potential side effects and risks. Most countries have some sort of government oversight organization that regulates drugs and medications. In the United States, this organization is the federal Food and Drug Administration (FDA). Only drugs that receive FDA approval can be marketed and sold in the United States. Although occasionally drugs have multiple approved uses, most have single and narrowly defined approved uses, and doctors must prescribe them accordingly.

Natural hormone support products are remedies, primarily derived from botanical (plant) sources, that you can buy without a prescription. Some are available in the form of teas or powders from crushed leaves, stems, or roots. Others are manufactured as concentrated extracts and are sold in tablets, capsules, liquids, and creams. Health food stores often carry the broadest selection of natural health products, although many grocery stores and retail pharmacies also sell them.

## Discussing Natural Hormone Support with Your Doctor

Always discuss your plans to use natural hormone support with your doctor, preferably before you start using them. This is particularly important if you're taking HRT or any other prescription medication on a regular basis. Some herbs contain substances that alter the way that other chemicals (such as drugs) work in your body (more on this later). Other herbal remedies could create problems for you if you have certain health conditions. If you're worried that your doctor will disapprove of your decision, it's time either for that heart-to-heart discussion you've been putting off or to choose a new physician who supports an integrative approach to healthcare.

Don't give up conventional, or allopathic, healthcare altogether, though. The essence of integrative care is to blend the best of all worlds, allopathic and complementary. Routine checkups are essential for catching potentially serious health concerns before they become problems. This gets more important as you grow older, especially if you have a family history of health conditions such as heart disease, osteoporosis, or breast, colon, or uterine cancer, or a personal history of a cervical abnormality such as dysplasia.

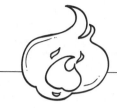

**Hot Flash!**

Don't let your enthusiasm for managing your own health get out of control. Self-treatment can be dangerous if you ignore the signs of potentially serious health problems. See your doctor for new signs and symptoms that stay around for longer than a couple of weeks, and for a regular checkup every year.

# Phytoestrogens: Estrogens from Plant Sources

Estrogens, as you remember from earlier chapters, are a group of chemical substances. The estrogens that your body produces belong to a chemical family called *steroidal estrogens*. The estrogens that plants make, *phytoestrogens,* belong to a chemically similar family called *phenolic estrogens*. The molecular structure of phenolic estrogens is similar to that of steroidal estrogens, which allows them to join in the same way with molecules in your body called estrogen receptors.

The differences in the rest of their molecular structures make phytoestrogens weaker than steroidal estrogens, and also alter the effects that phytoestrogens have on your body. Think of your body's hormone picture as a jigsaw puzzle. During meno-

**Wise Up**

**Steroidal estrogens** are the estrogens that your body produces. **Phytoestrogens** are the estrogens that plants make. *Phyto* is the Greek word for "plant." Phytoestrogens belong to a chemical family called **phenolic estrogens.**

pause, some puzzle pieces—your natural hormones—fall out of place. Phytoestrogens are like matching puzzle pieces cut out of paper: They fit into the space perfectly, but they're too thin to fill its depth.

Although there are few comprehensive research studies on phytoestrogens, most doctors believe that they are less effective than HRT in relieving menopause's discomforts and may not offer any long-term benefits. This is because phytoestrogens appear to have estrogenlike effects on some body systems but not on others. If this sounds familiar, think SERMs (selective estrogen receptor modulators). Researchers worked for many years to develop similar synthetic substances that could offer the benefits of estrogen replacement without the cancer risks. Some scientists believe that phytoestrogens could turn out to be nature's form of SERMs, although research studies to understand this facet of phytoestrogens are just getting underway.

There are dozens of phytoestrogens, which differ in their chemical structures. Four are the strongest and the most commonly used as menopause remedies: isoflavones, lignans, coumestans, and resorcyclic acid lactones. Many experts believe that the greatest benefit comes from consuming foods or taking supplements that contain all four of these groups of phytoestrogens. Here we'll present an overview of these substances. Chapters 19, "Soy, Herbs, and Other Botanicals: Nature's Menopause Miracles," and 20, "Nutrition: Eating Your Way Through a Healthy Menopause," discuss food and supplement sources for the different forms of phytoestrogens.

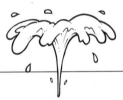

### Wellspring

In the 1940s, Australian sheep ranchers noticed an alarming drop in the number of pregnant ewes each spring. Before long, they linked the problem to the fields of clover they'd planted to provide a new source of food for their sheep—clover that was high in phytoestrogens. American and Canadian ranchers then began to question whether there was a correlation between food sources and fertility problems in cattle as well, even though their cattle weren't eating clover. They didn't have to search far for the answer: alfalfa. First-cut alfalfa hay proved to be extraordinarily high in phytoestrogens. In both situations, the estrogen effect was strong enough in the animals to function as natural birth contraception.

## Isoflavones

Isoflavones are a group of phytoestrogens that include genistein, daidzein, formononetin, biochanin, and glycitein. The strongest of the phytoestrogens, isoflavones, are still just one-hundredth to one-thousandth the strength of your body's natural estrogens. The foods with the highest concentrations of isoflavones are legumes, which include soybeans, chickpeas, clover, lentils, alfalfa, mung beans, lima beans, and black beans. Isoflavones appear to have cancer-preventing capabilities, especially against hormone-driven cancers such as breast cancer and uterine cancer. Isoflavones are also available in numerous supplement forms.

## Lignans

Whole grains (particularly wheat and rye), beans, vegetables, fruits, and flaxseeds contain phytoestrogens called lignans, with the highest concentrations found in flaxseeds. In addition to their estrogenlike effects, lignans appear to play a role in lowering cholesterol levels and in insulin sensitivity. A Finnish study identified a correlation between a high dietary intake of lignans and a lower breast cancer risk.

## Coumestans

Legumes—particularly soybeans, mung beans, clover, soy sprouts, and alfalfa sprouts—contain phytoestrogens called coumestans or coumesterols. Although coumestans don't produce as strong of an estrogen effect as isoflavones, some scientists theorize that coumestans and isoflavones in combination are more effective than either group of substances alone.

## Resorcyclic Acid Lactones

Resorcyclic acid lactones occur in grains such as rice, corn, barley, and wheat that are contaminated by a fungus. Because the fungus can be harmful in large quantities, most often this group of phytoestrogens is taken in the form of a supplement.

# The Safe Way to Use Natural Hormone Support

The benefits and risks of natural hormone support remain matters of debate among doctors and researchers. So how do you know what's safe and how to use it? A frank and open discussion with your gynecologist or women's healthcare specialist is a good place to start. This can help you identify any specific health concerns or problems that might affect your hormone support choices, alert you to potential complications or interactions, and steer you in the direction of reliable sources for supplements and herbal preparations.

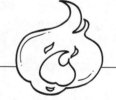

**Hot Flash!**

Don't combine natural hormone support with HRT unless your doctor tells you that it's okay to do so. Many botanical products can interfere with the actions of prescription hormone-replacement drugs.

Always follow the dosage recommendations on product labels, unless your doctor gives you other directions. If your discomforts don't improve after two or three weeks of using natural hormone support, see your doctor to be sure that there isn't something else going on. If you're following the guidance of an herbalist, you might need to fine-tune or revise your formulas and preparations.

## Identifying What You Need

Many women who use natural hormone support feel that they're on their own when it comes to identifying remedies to relieve their menopause discomforts. They move ahead on the basis of their signs and symptoms, and they make their way through a process of trial and error to find the remedies and products that do the job. Sometimes the process is short; sometimes it's not. The most ideal circumstance is to have an open and equitable partnership with your gynecologist or women's healthcare provider so that you can work together in this process.

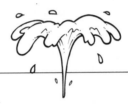

**Wellspring**

In an effort to help people evaluate the reality behind the testimonials and beliefs about what these products can do for you, the National Institutes of Health has established the National Center for Complementary and Alternative Medicine (NCCAM). According to its statement of purpose, the NCCAM "conducts and supports basic and applied research and training and disseminates information on complementary and alternative medicine to practitioners and the public." The NCCAM's Web site, www.nccam.nih.gov, is a quick and easy way to learn about what's new in complementary healthcare.

## Knowing What You're Getting

Most herbal and botanical preparations sold in the United States fall under the classification of food supplements when it comes to regulatory control. This means that they are not tested for efficacy (how well they work) or manufacturing consistency. As a result, there can be considerable variation in both for products that appear to be the same. Food supplements can make only generalized claims about their health benefits, and they don't have to list ingredients, risks, or side effects. These factors can make it challenging to figure out exactly what you're getting when you make a purchase. Here are some steps that you can take to know what you're getting when you buy herbal remedies:

➤ **Identify the preparation's active ingredients.** Most labels list the amount, either by measurement or by percentage, of the substances that are the botanical's active components. For example, chasteberry's active ingredient is agnuside.

➤ **Look for standardized extracts.** This means the product uses a manufacturing process that assures a consistent amount of active ingredient in each dosage form. This varies with the product. Chasteberry preparations, for example, should contain a standardized extract of 0.5 percent agnuside. Kava preparations should contain a standardized extract that is at least 30 percent kavalactones, the herb's active ingredient.

➤ **Determine the source of the extract.** Most herbalists believe that extracts from the plant's leaves, stems, or roots are more effective than purified extracts. Although this means that the preparation has a higher level of inactive ingredients, many herbalists feel that these add to the herb's effects. Purified extracts, on the other hand, are more highly processed. Think of it in terms of flour: Whole-wheat flour contains more particles of the grain, while white flour contains none. Both bake cakes, but the whole-wheat variety has added benefits such as fiber.

Above all, buy from reputable sources. Use brands that others recommend. Many doctors who are open to complementary therapies can recommend brands and products that they have come to trust, or that are solid from a pharmaceutical perspective.

## Choosing an Herbalist

An herbalist is someone—often a person trained in traditional Chinese medicine—who specializes in herbal remedies. Herbalists typically compound, or mix, preparations customized for your unique needs. However, there aren't any standard education, training, or licensing requirements for herbalists. Because herbs can be harmful if you use them incorrectly, it's important to find an herbalist who is knowledgeable and qualified. (One who is trained in traditional Chinese medicine has typically completed at least five years of education and practical experience.) If you want to go to an herbalist, ask for and contact references.

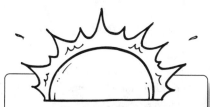

**Embracing Change**

As with other healthcare professionals, it's often helpful to get recommendations from trusted friends and family when you're looking for an herbalist. Interview several, if you can, to find one whose approach and philosophy are consistent with yours.

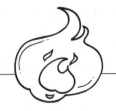

### Hot Flash!

Some combinations of herbs and botanicals can do more harm than good—and more is not necessarily better. Don't take more than the recommended dose, and learn all you can about the preparations that you want to take.

### Wise Woman's Wisdom

"Don't ever mind being called tough. Be strong and have definite ideas and opinions."

—Rosalyn Carter

## Foods or Supplements?

Most botanical remedies are easiest to purchase and use in supplement form. This includes powders, capsules, tablets, and liquids. You can mix them with foods or take them separately. Some herbal products really don't taste that great, so taking them as capsules or tablets gets around this and still gives you the active ingredients of the herbs. Some botanicals are available in the form of teas or can serve as seasonings in foods.

Many people believe that the closer to nature, the better. Others note that if an active ingredient's concentration is weak, you'd need to consume quite a quantity to get any benefit. Unfortunately, there aren't many studies to evaluate which is more effective. Often, it's a matter of personal preference. Some herbs are more effective in their natural state than as extracts, and others are more effective in the form of extracts. We'll discuss these in Chapter 19.

## Potential Complications and Interactions

It's easy to think that because you can buy a product literally anywhere, without a doctor's prescription, it must be "safe." This is a relative concept, however. Most products are safe for most people when taken according to the recommended doses. Taking more than you should, or taking the product more often than the directions specify, can have unpredictable and sometimes harmful consequences. If the product's label lists precautions or warnings, pay attention. If it's on the label, it has happened to more than just a few isolated individuals. For example, St. John's wort and dong quai increase your sensitivity to the sun's ultraviolet rays, making you more vulnerable to sunburn.

Interactions between natural remedies and prescription or over-the-counter medications that you take are also possible. Many herbal preparations, such as chasteberry and dong quai, relieve menopause discomforts by stimulating your body to increase its production of various "female" hormones. If you're also taking HRT, you could end up with hormone levels much higher than normal, creating a different set of problems for you. Herbal remedies can also interfere with medications prescribed to treat thyroid disease (hyperthyroidism and hypothyroidism), diabetes, high blood pressure, and depression. Do you have seasonal allergies or hay fever? If so, you might experience an allergic reaction to herbs such as chamomile, which is a member of the daisy family.

There's more about the potential complications and interactions of herbal remedies in Chapter 19.

# What If You Don't Take *Any* Hormones?

Most doctors believe that some sort of hormone support following menopause is better than none for most women. What that level of support should be to provide the optimal quality of life remains undetermined—and probably will vary according to individual health profiles and histories. In the short term, choosing not to take any hormones at all (neither HRT nor natural hormone supplements) might mean that hot flashes, mood swings, and irregular periods could be your companions for several years. During your transition through menopause, hormone supplements help relieve the discomforts that your body's fluctuating hormones cause.

After you've completed your menopause passage, hormone support serves an entirely different purpose. We're only now beginning to learn about the long-term effects of HRT as women reach their 70s, 80s, and beyond after having taken HRT. And we know more now than we did when Premarin reshaped the world's view of menopause back in the 1940s. Dosages today are much lower than they were in the early decades of HRT, and the variety of products available makes it possible to find an effective form of HRT for nearly every woman who wants to take it. Millions of women take or have taken HRT, providing a wealth of data for scientists to sort and evaluate.

The myriad of choices makes it more difficult for researchers to assess long-term risks as well as benefits, however. Most studies have looked at HRT in general and without distinguishing among the various forms and doses that women take. Do estrogen pills have the same benefits and risks as estrogen patches, for example? Does one formulation of estrogens have the same effect as another? Doctors have always assumed so, although this is far from certain. It is clear that future studies of HRT and natural hormone support will address, and even focus on, many of these finer points. Doctors also hope that future studies will pinpoint the precise role of HRT in heart disease, osteoporosis, and cancer, providing a better understanding of benefits and risks.

## The Least You Need to Know

➤ Natural doesn't mean risk-free. Natural hormone support is a therapeutic approach that requires careful assessment and regular oversight.

➤ Although the likelihood of unpleasant side effects is much lower with natural hormone support than with HRT, it's possible that the benefits are less significant as well.

➤ Phytoestrogens are similar to the estrogens your body produces, but they are weaker and chemically different.

➤ Always let your gynecologist know what herbal remedies or botanical preparations you're taking, and be sure that you understand their potential risks and side effects.

➤ Buy standardized supplements from reputable manufacturers. In the United States, most natural hormone support products are considered food supplements and are not subject to the rigorous testing that drugs must go through.

# Chapter 19

# Soy, Herbs, and Other Botanicals: Nature's Menopause Miracles

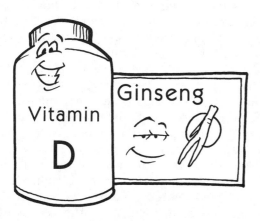

## In This Chapter

➤ Why soy is the magical bean

➤ How estrogen receptors work

➤ How to increase the soy in your diet

➤ How traditional Chinese herbs can relieve your menopause discomforts

➤ Other herbs and plant products that can ease your journey through menopause

In the quest for safer alternatives to HRT, many women have turned to substances found in nature. Many herbal remedies and botanical preparations claim to ease the discomforts of menopause. And many women do find relief in using these therapies, at least in the short term.

What concerns doctors more is what happens in the long term, with hormone-related conditions such as osteoporosis. Can botanicals help there? Surprisingly, new research shows that certain plants might contain substances that protect your bones—and also help protect against cancer and heart disease.

# Is It True, No Hot Flashes with Soy?

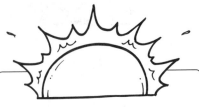

**Embracing Change**

Hot flashes are so uncommon among Japanese women that there is no native Japanese word for them.

As media reports in recent years have presented it, soy is the magical bean. It prevents cancer, lowers cholesterol and your risk for heart disease, and nearly extinguishes hot flashes. Can one substance truly do so much good? The answer may well be a qualified "yes." Soy—or, more specifically, soy isoflavones—do seem to have amazing health benefits. Researchers have known for years, for example, that people living in countries such as Japan, where soy foods are part of every meal, are significantly less likely to get a variety of health conditions, including heart disease and certain cancers. We also know that far fewer women in these countries experience hot flashes, mood swings, and other discomforts of menopause. Although clearly there are a number of lifestyle factors that affect health, researchers have finally zeroed in on the role of soy. What they've recently discovered may unlock an entirely new approach to hormone support.

**Wise Up**

**Estrogen receptors** are the protein molecules within the body's tissue cells that connect to the molecules in estrogens.

## *Estrogen Receptors: Completing the Connection*

The molecules that form the basic chemical structure of estrogen connect with (or bind to, in more scientific terms) protein molecules in body tissue cells called *estrogen receptors*. The effect is like plugging in a lamp. When estrogen "plugs" into a cell's estrogen receptors, it affects genes within the cell that are sensitive to the connection. This causes the cell to take certain actions. Going back to our lamp analogy, the light bulb would light up or turn off, depending on its state before the connection took place. If the activated cell is in your ovary, it could begin the process of ripening an egg. If it's in your breast and you're pregnant, it could begin the process of making milk. And in bone tissue, the activated cell could block the release of calcium, while an unactivated cell could allow your body to drain calcium from your bones, weakening them and setting the stage for osteoporosis.

Researchers have known about estrogen receptors for decades. They've also known that some tissues in your body have more estrogen receptors than other tissues, making those tissues estrogen-sensitive. But they only recently discovered that there are at least two (and presumably more) kinds of estrogen receptors. Suddenly there was an objective and scientific explanation for how estrogen has different effects not only in different tissues but also in different people. (Picture a light bulb glowing over their heads!) In the methodical, though less-than-creative, manner of science, this second kind of estrogen receptor was named ER beta (the Greek word for "two" or "second"). And because there were now at least two ERs, the first was renamed ER alpha (the Greek word for "one" or "first").

The discovery of ER beta helped clear up the mystery what role estrogen plays in conditions such as osteoporosis. (It also paved the way for the development of synthetic SERMs.) Although bone cells don't have much ER alpha, they have an abundance of ER beta. Steroidal estrogens, such as those in HRT and your body's natural hormones, bind to both kinds of estrogen receptors. Isoflavones, the phytoestrogens found in soy and other plants, form only a weak connection with ER alpha (like plugging in a cord that has only one prong). But they connect with ER beta with nearly the same strength as steroidal hormones. This might explain why women whose diets are high in soy escape both the discomforts of menopause and the risk of serious health problems such as cancer and heart disease. Even though they receive hormone replacement through the soy products they eat, the phytoestrogens bond only with ER beta. Researchers are now studying the correlation between cancer and the extended activation of ER alpha by the steroidal estrogens in HRT.

## Soy Isoflavones

Isoflavones are the most active and abundant phytoestrogens found in soy. Some forms of soy contain higher concentrations of isoflavones than others. Generally, the less the soy is processed, the more isoflavones it contains. Products such as soy burgers and soy hotdogs provide only moderate amounts of isoflavones. Highly processed soy products such as soy sauce and soy oil don't have any isoflavones at all.

People in Japan consume the highest concentrations of soy isoflavones through the foods they eat, around 200 milligrams (mg) a day. People in other cultures, in which soy products are common, may eat about a fourth of that, or about 50 mg a day. People in the West, and particularly the United States, typically consume less than 5 mg of soy isoflavones a day. Most health experts recommend at least 50 mg of soy isoflavones a day to ease the discomforts of menopause.

## The Myriad of Soy Benefits for Your General Health

Many health experts have long suspected that soy reduces cholesterol levels and thus lowers your risk for heart disease. In the 1990s, scientific studies established evidence supporting this. It appears that soy protein, rather than soy isoflavones, gets the credit for this effect. Other studies continue to explore the links between soy and cancer, osteoporosis, food allergies, diabetes, and kidney disease. Soy is an excellent source of protein, making it a nutritious, low-fat substitute for meat.

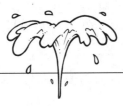

**Wellspring**

The FDA recommends that adults consume 25 mg of soy protein a day to lower blood cholesterol levels and reduce the risk of heart disease. Many products that are high in soy protein are low in soy isoflavones, however. If you're using soy to both control your cholesterol and to reduce your menopause discomforts, be sure that you know what you're getting. For example, soy protein concentrate is high in soy proteins and is easy to add to just about any food. But it may contain little or no isoflavones, depending on how it is manufactured. Soy isolate powder and soy flour, on the other hand, contain high concentrations of isoflavones. If in doubt, contact the product's manufacturer for its complete nutritional content. Most package labels don't include this information.

**Wise Up**

**Legumes** are plants that produce fruits or seeds that humans can eat. The word *legume* comes from the Latin word *legere,* which means "to gather." Beans and peas are the most common legumes.

# How to Get Soy in Your Diet—and Like It

If soy is so good for you, why aren't you eating all you can? Well, soybeans aren't exactly appealing. Rather bland in flavor and appearance, straight soybeans are an acquired taste. Like other *legumes,* soybeans must be cooked in some fashion before humans can eat and digest them. They have tough outer skins that, if uncooked, even digestive acids can't penetrate. And even eating cooked soybeans can have, shall we say, noticeable digestive consequences (gas!). So, the challenge has been to create ways of using soybeans in ways that make them more appetizing.

Soy products such as tofu and tempeh are becoming increasingly popular because they can be easy and tasty meat and dairy replacements in a variety of dishes, dips, and dressings. If you like traditional bean sprouts, try soybean sprouts instead. Burgers made from textured soy protein aren't as high in soy isoflavones as other soy products, but they're more popular with people who enjoy the texture and flavor of traditional meat burgers. And if you can't stomach the thought of soy-based foods at all, supplements in capsule or powder form can add soy isoflavones to your diet without changing your favorite recipes.

## Common Soy Foods

| Food Product | Serving Size (Approximate) | Isoflavone Content Per Serving |
|---|---|---|
| Boiled soybeans | ½ cup | 150 mg |
| Roasted soybeans | ½ cup | 170 mg |
| Soy flour | ½ cup | 45 mg |
| Soy grits | ¼ cup | 45 mg |
| Soy isolate powder | 1 oz. | 60 mg |
| Soymilk | 1 cup | 20 mg |
| Tempeh | 4 oz. | 60 mg |
| Textured soy protein | ½ cup | 55 mg (dry) |
| Tofu | 4 oz. | 40 mg |

# Other Sources for Phytoestrogens

Although soy gets the lion's share of credit for supplying us with phytoestrogens, it's not the only source of these valuable natural substances. In fact, nearly all fruits and vegetables contain some concentration of phytoestrogens.

## Not Just for Rabbits: Red Clover

Soy products may be gradually infiltrating the Western diet, but not many people are drinking red clover tea. If your menopause transition has gotten a bit bumpy, though, you might want to give it a try. Soy's two primary phytoestrogens are the isoflavones genistein and daidzein. Red clover contains these, as well as two others with strong, estrogenlike actions, formonoetin and biochanin. Red clover also contains other phytoestrogens called coumestans. Preliminary research suggests that coumestans might be up to six times stronger than other phytoestrogens.

Usually taken in tea form, red clover is a popular herbal remedy in many cultures. In some women, red clover appears to be more effective than soy in relieving menopause discomforts such as hot flashes, although it's not as effective as HRT. Red clover extract forms the basis of a product called Promensil, manufactured and marketed by a company called Novagen.

## Peas, Lentils, and Other Legumes

If it comes in a pod, it's a seed and it contains phytoestrogens. The seed is the ovum, or egg, of the plant and is naturally high in plant estrogens. Eating plenty of legumes other than soybeans can help you get a weak but steady supply of phytoestrogens. Other common legumes include peas, lima beans, black beans, and lentils. Alfalfa sprouts are particularly high in coumestans.

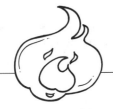

**Hot Flash!**

Some traditional Chinese herbs contain powerful chemicals that, if mixed together improperly, can be harmful. If you want to use these remedies, be sure to obtain them from experienced herbalists.

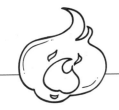

**Hot Flash!**

Do not take dong quai if you're taking prescription anticoagulants (blood-thinners) or aspirin. Also stop taking it at least two weeks before any scheduled surgery, and be sure to let your surgeon know that you've been taking it. Dong quai has a mild anticoagulant action.

# Traditional Chinese Herbs

The remedies of traditional Chinese medicine (TCM) date back at least 2,500 years and probably further. This approach to health and healing views the body as an integrated and balanced system that is itself an element in the larger natural environment. TCM views disease as an imbalance of the body's life energy, or chi. Remedies emphasize restoring this balance. Most feature blends of various herbs and other botanicals to provide a broad therapeutic base. A few achieve specific results when taken individually. Traditional Chinese herbs are most often sold or mixed fresh or dried, and may be less effective in supplement form.

Unlike soy and other legumes, traditional Chinese herbs do not contain phytoestrogens. Some have what scientists call estrogenic, or estrogenlike, actions in the body. Others are not well enough understood to know their actions. Most experts believe it's difficult to isolate the active ingredients in herbs, and suspect that it's the herbs' ingredients in combination with one another that give them their therapeutic abilities. Although traditional Chinese herbs are used by many cultures around the world, there are few clinical studies of them.

## Dong Quai (Angelica)

Prepared from the root of the flowering plant known scientifically as *Angelica sinensis,* dong quai is a remedy for hot flashes, vaginal dryness, and irregular bleeding. Herbalists often prescribe it as a general tonic to improve the functioning of the reproductive system overall. In TCM, dong quai is usually boiled and served as a tea, but many Western women prefer to take an extract of this herb in capsule form. Different varieties of Angelica herbs exist, so read the label to be sure that you're getting the right one.

Dong quai often appears in herbal blends sold as menopause remedies that may contain Siberian ginseng, black cohosh, chasteberry, kava, and dandelion root. Certain chemicals in dong quai increase sensitivity to ultraviolet sunlight, so use sunscreen and wear protective clothing when you're outside.

# Ginseng (Panax)

Nearly a dozen varieties of ginseng exist. The one used in TCM is Chinese ginseng, known scientifically as *Panax ginseng*. In TCM, ginseng is often used as a general tonic to bring balance to a particular body system or the body as a whole by restoring chi. Ginseng stimulates the adrenal glands, which in turn affects the body's production of various hormones including estrogen and progesterone. Ginseng has a reputation for increasing vitality and sex drive in both men and women.

Not all ginseng products—including ginseng roots—are equal. The ginseng root's active ingredients are substances called ginsenosides. It takes 6 to 10 years for the root to contain enough ginsenosides to have any therapeutic effect. It's nearly impossible to measure the level of ginsenosides in roots, of course, making it especially important to buy them from a reputable source. Products containing Chinese ginseng extract should contain at least 2 percent ginsenosides.

Because of ginseng's estrogenic effects, you shouldn't use it without your doctor's approval if you're taking HRT or birth control pills, or if you could be pregnant. American ginseng (*Panax quinquefolium*) and Siberian ginseng (*Eleutherococcus senticosis*) have similar but less pronounced effects.

# Motherwort

This herb's Chinese name translates into English as "good mother herb." TCM uses motherwort for a variety of menstrual and menopausal symptoms, including irregular bleeding, cramps, and fluid retention. Some tests suggest that motherwort can help the uterus contract after giving birth. Chinese pharmacies and some health food stores sell fresh, dried, or powdered motherwort leaves and stems. Herbalists often blend motherwort with other herbs.

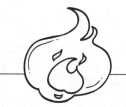

**Hot Flash!**

Do not use motherwort if you could be pregnant. Its ability to cause uterine contractions can result in miscarriages.

# Other Helping Herbs and Botanicals

Many plant-based remedies for the discomforts of menopause don't contain any form of estrogen or other hormones. Instead, they induce biochemical reactions in your body that affect its hormone production. Although these remedies have been used in various cultures for many years (often centuries), there are few scientific studies to corroborate their therapeutic claims. It often takes several weeks to several months of consistent use for many herbal remedies to take effect.

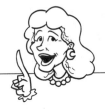

# Black Cohosh

Black cohosh (*Cimicifuga racemosa*) comes from the root of a wildflower that originated in the American plains. A favorite of Native American women in centuries past, today black cohosh is the leading herbal remedy sold in Europe to treat the discomforts of menopause. Its primary therapeutic value is relieving hot flashes and vaginal dryness. Although its actions in the human body haven't been well studied, black cohosh appears to function in an estrogenlike way, perhaps mildly stimulating the ovaries to increase estrogen production somewhat. This botanical has a wider variation of results among women who take it, as do botanicals high in phytoestrogens (such as soy and red clover).

The primary active ingredients appear to be triterpene glycosides, although most herbalists believe that other ingredients are also important even though they haven't yet been isolated. Women who experience the best results with black cohosh take a preparation that uses freeze-dried root, either in capsules or prepared as tea. Black cohosh extract also comes in liquid form. Freeze-dried black cohosh should contain at least 2.5 percent triterpene glycosides, while liquid forms should contain at least 5 percent.

Because black cohosh has estrogenic effects, consult with your doctor first if you're already taking HRT or birth control pills.

# Chasteberry (Vitex)

Chasteberries (*Vitex agnus-castus*) come from the chaste tree, which grows in the Mediterranean region. The reddish-brown berries look and taste like peppercorns and are sometimes called monk's pepper. When consumed, chasteberries act on the pituitary gland, stimulating it to release luteinizing hormone (LH) and to cut back on prolactin. The increase in LH causes the ovaries to produce more progesterone. This result helps relieve hot flashes, sleep disturbances, and vaginal dryness. In some women, chasteberry improves mood swings, although in other women irritability can worsen.

Chasteberry preparations are available as powders for tea, capsules, and liquids. Extracts should be standardized to 0.5 percent. Because chasteberry causes progesterone levels to increase, it can cause increased flow if you're still having periods. Chasteberry is commonly included in blended preparations. As with other estrogenic botanicals, check with your doctor if you're already taking HRT or birth control pills.

# Damiana

Damiana is an herb reputed to have *aphrodisiac* qualities. Some herbalists believe that damiana has little or no therapeutic value, while others feel that it stimulates testosterone production to increase sex drive and overall energy. There are no scientific studies to support or refute either position. Damiana sometimes is included in combination products for treating menopause discomforts, and is available in tea and capsule forms.

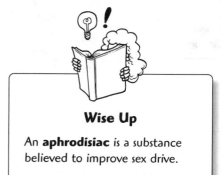

**Wise Up**

An **aphrodisiac** is a substance believed to improve sex drive.

# Dandelion Root

Those yellow blobs in the green sea of your lawn mark the location of what might be considered nature's drug store: the dandelion. The root and leaves of this perennial pest contain dozens of vitamins and chemicals that foster good health. The functions of these substances are more general than menopause-specific. Herbalists may recommend various dandelion preparations to treat fluid retention, tender breasts, inflamed joints, constipation, fever, and other health concerns.

# Evening Primrose Oil

Evening primrose oil contains the fatty acids linoleic acid and gammalinolenic acid. As a menopause remedy, evening primrose oil sometimes helps with discomforts such as breast tenderness (and is also used in PMS for the same purpose). Many herbalists use this substance as a tonic for general health, particularly during times of physical and emotional stress.

# Sage

Perhaps more familiar as a Thanksgiving seasoning, sage can calm hot flashes and sleep disturbances during menopause. This common herb, which is easy to grow yourself, has estrogenic actions in the body. Herbalists most often prescribe sage in the form of tea, although powder and liquid extracts are available and appear to be just as effective. Sage contains numerous active ingredients including thujones, camphor, triterpenes, steroids, flavones, flavonoids, and glycosides.

## Common Botanical Remedies for the Discomforts of Menopause

| For This Discomfort ... | Try ... |
| --- | --- |
| Breast tenderness | Evening primrose oil, dandelion root, motherwort |
| Fluid retention | Dandelion root, motherwort |
| Hot flashes | Soy isoflavones, red clover, black cohosh, chasteberry, wild yam, sage, dong quai, ginseng |
| Irregular periods | Motherwort, dong quai, chasteberry |
| Irritability and mood swings | Chasteberry, gingko, St. John's wort, wild yam |
| Lack of energy or sex drive | Ginseng, gingko, damiana, wild yam |
| Sleep disturbances | Kava, valerian, chasteberry, sage, chamomile |
| Vaginal dryness | Wild yam (especially cream), black cohosh, dong quai, chasteberry |

# Feeling Better ... Naturally

Some herbal remedies target your overall sense of well-being, aiding with such generalized problems as low energy, sleep disturbances, tension due to stress, and mild depression. Often preparations marketed as menopause remedies include small amounts of these herbs in their combinations.

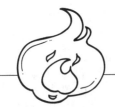

**Hot Flash!**

Many herbs—including ginkgo and ginseng—have blood-thinning effects. Talk with your doctor about taking any herbs or complementary remedies if you're regularly taking aspirin or other anticoagulants.

## Chamomile

Chamomile is a gentle sedative and a smooth muscle relaxant most commonly taken as tea. In addition to creating a sense of relaxation, chamomile eases menstrual cramps by helping to relax the smooth muscle tissue of the uterus. Chamomile is available in many forms. Most people enjoy the pleasant, applelike aroma and flavor of the tea, which is usually brewed from the plant's dried flowers. Chamomile is a member of the daisy family and can cause reactions similar to hay fever in people who have seasonal allergies.

## Gingko Biloba

Gingko trees have survived droughts, fires, ice ages, and even the atomic bomb that fell on Hiroshima. An individual tree can live for 1,000 years. It's not surprising that from this enduring life form come a number of healing remedies. Gingko's ability to improve circulation at the capillary level (the body's smallest blood vessels) is credited with this botanical's many therapeutic effects. Some scientists believe that if there is a fountain of youth, it flows from the ginkgo tree.

Herbalists prescribe ginkgo to treat memory loss; senility; chronic circulatory disorders, including Reynaud's syndrome, a painful condition in which circulation to the hands and feet is very poor, leaving them cold and bluish; tinnitus, ringing of the ears; and vertigo, chronic dizziness. Ginkgo is available in the form of dried leaves for making tea, as well as in powder and liquid extracts. Most extracts contain flavonoids, the most prominent of gingko's numerous active ingredients. Herbalists generally recommend that you start with a lower dose of gingko and build up to a therapeutic dose to avoid developing headaches.

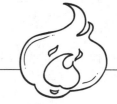

**Hot Flash!**

Depression can be a serious condition that requires medical attention. It's always a good idea to see your doctor before you start treating yourself, if for no other reason than to be sure that there's not an underlying medical cause·for your symptoms. If you start taking St. John's wort and don't notice any improvement in a month or so, contact your doctor.

## Kava

Kava, also called kava kava (*Piper methysticum*), is a member of the pepper family that is native to the South Seas islands of Micronesia, Polynesia, and Melanesia. Although its active ingredients haven't been identified, kava is becoming popular for its mild sedative and muscle-relaxant effects. Extracts typically contain kavalactones, although several studies have shown that kavalactones alone don't have the same effect as a preparation that uses the whole root. Low doses taken during the day help relieve anxiety, while a higher dose taken before bedtime aids in falling asleep.

Taking too much kava can make you feel intoxicated. Unlike alcohol intoxication, however, kava intoxication creates a sense of deep relaxation and well-being right before you fall asleep.

## St. John's Wort (Hypericum)

Known as nature's antidepressant, St. John's wort is so called because it blooms around June 23, which is St. John's Eve. (*Wort* means "herb.") The plant's leaves "bleed" a red oil when crushed. This oil, found in the bright yellow flowers as well,

**215**

has several active ingredients, including the glucoside hypericin and various flavo-noids. St. John's wort, or *Hypericum perforatum* as it's known scientifically, is the most commonly prescribed antidepressant in Europe. Studies show that hypericin has a direct effect on the neurotransmitters that regulate mood, similar to action of prescription drugs called selective serotonin reuptake inhibitors (such as Prozac and Zoloft).

## Valerian

Valerian is becoming increasingly popular as a mild and effective sleep aid. It shortens the amount of time that it takes to fall asleep, and it helps you sleep for longer periods without waking. It doesn't appear to interrupt dream patterns or have any sort of "hangover" effect (when you feel groggy and out of touch the next morning). Fresh or dried root are the preferred forms for brewing tea. Extracts in capsule form should contain 0.8 percent valeric acid, the herb's active ingredient. Using valerian every night for longer than two or three weeks can result in headaches, however, and the herb's effectiveness may become reduced.

Don't use valerian if you're taking any other sleep aids, and talk with your doctor first if you're taking medication to regulate your blood pressure (valerian can lower blood pressure). Valerian root has a strong, rather pungent odor.

## Wild Yam: Natural Progesterone?

Wild, or Mexican, yams contain substances that are important precursors (building blocks) for progesterone. The two most active of these are diosgenin and seponin, which stimulate your body's adrenal glands to increase production of progesterone. Wild yams do not actually contain progesterone, although they do contain mild phytoestrogens. Wild yam extract is especially popular in cream form, which, when applied to various skin surfaces, is absorbed into your body in a process similar to wearing a progesterone patch.

# Giving Natural Remedies the Respect They Deserve

Just because something's natural doesn't mean it's without risk. Herbs and other botanicals can have powerful effects, and can have potentially hazardous interactions when you mix them together. If you want to use herbal remedies, stay with prepared combinations or try to find a qualified herbalist or traditional Chinese medicine (TCM) practitioner who can guide you. Always—and we can't stress this enough—tell your primary care physician what you're taking. If your doctor disapproves of complementary therapies, find a doctor who shares your views and has the knowledge to help you develop an integrative treatment approach that's right for your health needs.

## The Least You Need to Know

➤ Although herbs and botanical preparations are generally safe, they can interact with other substances or each other to produce harmful side effects.

➤ Soy has numerous health benefits beyond its ability to relieve the discomforts of menopause, including protection against heart disease and cancer.

➤ Obtain herbal remedies from a trusted source or an experienced herbalist. This helps assure that you'll get the correct dose and strength.

➤ Try combination herbal remedies for the broadest therapeutic benefits.

➤ Botanical preparations that have estrogenic effects can interfere with HRT and birth control pills.

➤ Consult with your doctor about herbal remedies that you're considering. This is especially important if you're already taking HRT or other prescription or over-the-counter medications.

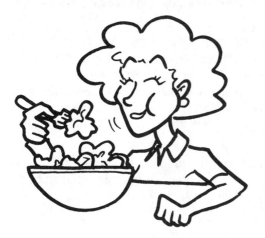

# Chapter 20

# Nutrition: Eating Your Way Through a Healthy Menopause

---

### In This Chapter

➤ What it means to eat right for a healthy menopause

➤ Identifying when and how much you eat: a self-quiz

➤ Calculating your body mass index (BMI)

➤ Managing your weight the healthy way

➤ Making nutritious food choices

➤ How to get the vitamins and minerals that your body needs during menopause

---

Are your eating habits filling your body with empty calories? Many of us eat on the run, grabbing what's fast and easy in between the events of our busy lives. Although you can get a burger and fries at any time nearly anywhere you happen to be, trying to find fresh vegetables and fruits can be a challenge.

Healthy choices aren't always easy to make. Some experts believe that many people who believe that they eat nutritiously still short-change their bodies. And people who pay little attention to nutritional content actually could have deficiencies of key vitamins and minerals.

# Are You Eating Right for a Healthy Menopause?

In many respects, eating right for a healthy menopause is no different than eating right for a healthy life. Balance and moderation are the operative concepts. However, your nutritional needs are changing, as is your body's metabolism. By age 50, your body uses 150 fewer calories a day than it did 20 or 30 years earlier. But you've become accustomed to eating at the level that sustained your body all these years, and there's no red warning light that starts flashing when your body's nutritional tank is full. Your body simply converts those extra calories into fat, storing them for future use.

Unless you increase your level of physical activity to compensate, those extra calories will total 54,750 by year's end, translating into more than 15 pounds of added body weight! So don't just sit there—take action. Make a walk before meals a part of your routine. You'll eat less, and your metabolism will be higher to help put what you do eat to good use.

## What and How Much Do You Eat? A Self-Quiz

Do you make nutritious choices when it's time to feed your appetite? Even people who think that they do are often surprised to find out that they really don't. Here are a few questions to help you assess your eating habits. Be honest, now!

1. I usually eat when …
   a. It's mealtime.
   b. I'm stressed, it's the week before my period, or someone's celebrating something.
   c. Everyone else has gone to bed.
   d. I feel hungry.

2. I choose what foods to eat based on …
   a. Whether they come chocolate-coated.
   b. What I can buy with the change I have.
   c. What's in the fridge.
   d. Their food group and nutritional content.

3. A serving size is …
   a. Whatever it takes to fill my plate.
   b. However much I can eat before I have to be somewhere or do something.
   c. Bigger for foods that stack and smaller for foods that spread out on the plate, so more looks like less.
   d. Whatever it takes to make me feel full.

**4.** I know it's time to stop eating when …

    **a.** I notice that other people are staring at me.

    **b.** I'd have to fix more food to keep eating.

    **c.** I look at my plate and feel guilty.

    **d.** I feel full.

**5.** My favorite snack is …

    **a.** Anything chocolate.

    **b.** Anything salty.

    **c.** A "good" food and a "bad" food, like bananas sliced over ice cream or carrots with ranch dip.

    **d.** An apple, a handful of raisins, and some roasted soy nuts.

So are you eating as well as you thought? If three or more of your answers are Ds, you're probably doing a pretty good job of meeting your body's nutritional needs. If most of your answers are As, Bs, or Cs, congratulations on your honesty and your sense of adventure—but you'd better sit up straight and take notes. Your food choices likely are too often less than nutritious, and you'll soon be paying the price if you don't make some changes.

# Poor Nutrition and (Over)Weight

Being overweight is a serious health risk for many medical conditions that become more common at midlife and beyond, such as diabetes, heart disease (including high blood pressure and stroke), cancer, and osteoporosis. Public health officials estimate that about 60 percent of American adults weigh at least 20 percent more than they should. Extra weight makes your body work harder in nearly every aspect of its functions. Although in our culture we tend to focus on the appearance issues of being overweight, it's what you *can't* see that can do you the greatest harm. There is some evidence, however, that women who are overweight have fewer discomforts during menopause. Researchers believe that this is because fat cells produce small amounts of estrogen.

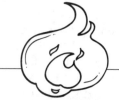

**Hot Flash!**

Eating disorders affect women of all ages and backgrounds. If you have trouble controlling your eating habits because you either eat too much or too little, seek professional help. Your health—and your life—could be at risk.

Being underweight can be a health concern, too. Women who are shorter than 5 feet, 4 inches in height and who have slight builds are at increased risk for osteoporosis. Being significantly underweight can also compromise your immune system and alter your hormone balance, especially if your weight approaches the zone in which your

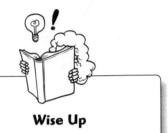

**Wise Up**

Your **body mass index** (**BMI**) is a mathematical calculation that categorizes your risk for health problems as it relates to your body weight.

body interprets your situation to be one of starvation. It begins to shut down nonessential functions, including the hormone cycles that regulate menstruation. This increases the state of confusion that your body is in and makes it less likely that you'll receive relief from menopause remedies that would otherwise be helpful.

## How Much Should You Weigh?

The weight that's ideal for your body is the one that supports its nutritional and functional needs to create an environment of health and wellness. In general, this is a weight that's in proportion to your height, and it may drift a few pounds in either direction.

Before the 1990s, doctors used the dreaded height and weight charts to determine whether you were tall enough to justify your weight. We dreaded these charts not just because they reduced the challenges of weight control to a mark that fell either between the lines (yea!) or beyond the lines (groan). The charts were also hard to follow, and they failed to consider factors such as muscle mass. You could have a small, medium, or large frame—and a different weight range for each.

Now there's a more precise assessment tool called the *body mass index,* better known as *BMI.* BMI uses a mathematical formula to calculate the relationship between your weight, your height, and other factors, such as muscle mass. Ready for today's math lesson? Your BMI is your weight in kilograms divided by your height in meters squared, or $BMI = kg/m^2$. Your answer, or index, identifies your relative risk of developing health problems related to obesity. The National Institutes of Health has assigned health risk categories to BMI ranges.

## Body Mass Index (BMI) Health Risk Scale

| If Your BMI Is ... | Then Your Health Risk Status Is ... |
| --- | --- |
| 18.5 or under | Underweight, with possible health risks |
| 18.6 to 24.9 | Normal, with average health risks |
| 25.0 to 27.9 | Overweight, with increased health risks |
| 28.0 to 39.9 | Obese, with very high health risks |
| 40 or over | Extremely obese, with extremely high health risks |

Here's how to calculate your BMI. You'll need a scale, a measuring tape, and a calculator.

1. Take off all your clothes and weigh yourself on an accurate scale.

   My weight is _____ pounds.

2. Put your clothes back on (except your shoes) if you like, and get a calculator. Multiply your weight in pounds by .45 to convert to kilograms.

   My weight in kilograms is _____ kg.

3. Stand against a wall in your bare feet, heels to the wall. Have someone measure your height, and then convert the measurement to inches.

   My height is _____ feet, _____ inches.

   My height in inches is _____ inches.

4. Multiply your height in inches by .025 (this converts it to meters), and then multiply the result by itself (this squares it).

   My height in meters is _____ meters.

   My height in meters squared is _____ $m^2$.

5. Divide your weight in kilograms by your height in meters squared. The answer is your BMI.

   My weight in kilograms (_____ kg) divided by my height in meters squared (_____ $m^2$) is _____.

6. Locate your BMI range on the table showing the BMI Health Risk Scale. This is your health risk status.

   My BMI is _____, which gives me a health risk status of _____.

Confused? Here's an example. Say that you weigh 150 pounds and you're 5 feet 4 inches tall. Your weight in kilograms is 67.5 kg ($150 \times .45 = 67.5$). Your height in inches is 64 inches ($5 \times 12 = 60 + 4 = 64$), which is 1.6 meters ($64 \times .025 = 1.625$). Multiply this number by itself to square it, and you get 2.56 $m^2$. When you divide your weight in kilograms (67.5) by your height in meters squared (2.56), you get 26.36. Rounded to 26.4, this is overweight with an increased risk of health problems. You can see, however, that losing just 10 pounds drops your health risk back within the average range.

# Meeting Your Nutritional Needs Through the Foods You Eat

Many experts believe that most healthy adults *can* meet their nutritional needs through the foods they eat, if they choose their foods with nutrition in mind. Whether they succeed or not is a more complex question. In today's fast-paced world, that's sometimes more fantasy than reality. To help people translate good nutrition into wise food choices, the USDA has developed a simple chart called the Food Guide Pyramid. This chart shows how many servings of what foods you should eat each day

to meet your body's nutritional needs; turn back to Chapter 13, "Sexuality, Those 10 Extra Pounds, and Menopause," to take another look at the USDA Food Guide Pyramid.

Many processed foods such as cereals and breads are fortified with vitamins and minerals to help you meet your body's daily nutritional requirements. The FDA requires all packaged foods sold in the United States to list the product's ingredients and nutritional content on the product's label. The label shows the nutrient's quantity as well as the percentage of the *daily values* (*DVs*) that it provides. Other food products contain added vitamins and minerals that they don't have in their natural states. For example, many brands of orange juice are fortified with vitamin D and calcium.

If you could eat foods entirely as they exist in nature, would you meet your body's nutritional requirements? Today's farming practices make this less of a certainty than it was 50 or 100 years ago. Thanks to fertilization and technology, farmland may support several cycles of crops in a year. This draws steadily from the nutrients that come from the soil. Crops, including fruits and vegetables, may not be as nutrient-dense as you expect them to be. As well, modern harvesting methods typically involve picking fruits and vegetables just before they fully ripen to extend their freshness in the stores. To counter these factors, many people choose produce and grains grown organically—without added fertilizers, ripening agents, or preservatives.

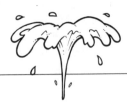

# Nutrition Facts

Serving Size 1 cup (30g)
Servings Per Container About 14

| Amount Per Serving | Cheerios | with ½ cup skim milk |
|---|---|---|
| **Calories** | 110 | 150 |
| Calories from Fat | 15 | 20 |
| | **% Daily Value**** | |
| **Total Fat** 2g* | **3%** | **3%** |
| Saturated Fat 0g | **0%** | **3%** |
| Polyunsaturated Fat 0.5g | | |
| Monounsaturated Fat 0.5g | | |
| **Cholesterol** 0mg | **0%** | **1%** |
| **Sodium** 280mg | **12%** | **15%** |
| **Potassium** 95mg | **3%** | **9%** |
| **Total Carbohydrate** 22g | **7%** | **9%** |
| Dietary Fiber 3g | **11%** | **11%** |
| Soluble Fiber 1g | | |
| Sugars 1g | | |
| Other Carbohydrate 18g | | |
| **Protein** 3g | | |
| Vitamin A | 10% | 15% |
| Vitamin C | 10% | 10% |
| Calcium | 4% | 20% |
| Iron | 45% | 45% |
| Vitamin D | 10% | 25% |
| Thiamin | 25% | 30% |
| Riboflavin | 25% | 35% |
| Niacin | 25% | 25% |
| Vitamin $B_6$ | 25% | 25% |
| Folic Acid | 25% | 25% |
| Vitamin $B_{12}$ | 25% | 35% |
| Phosphorus | 10% | 25% |
| Magnesium | 8% | 10% |
| Zinc | 25% | 30% |
| Copper | 2% | 2% |

*Amount in Cereal. A serving of cereal plus skim milk provides 2g fat (0.5g saturated fat, 1g monounsaturated fat), less than 5mg cholesterol, 350mg sodium, 300mg potassium, 28g carbohydrate (7g sugars) and 7g protein.

**Percent Daily Values are based on a 2,000 calorie diet. Your daily values may be higher or lower depending on your calorie needs:

| | Calories: | 2,000 | 2,500 |
|---|---|---|---|
| Total Fat | Less than | 65g | 80g |
| Sat Fat | Less than | 20g | 25g |
| Cholesterol | Less than | 300mg | 300mg |
| Sodium | Less than | 2,400mg | 2,400mg |
| Potassium | | 3,500mg | 3,500mg |
| Total Carbohydrate | | 300g | 375g |
| Dietary Fiber | | 25g | 30g |

*Here's a food label from a whole-grain oat cereal.*

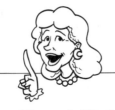

# Here a Diet, There a Diet, Everywhere You Look a Diet

Doctors and nutritionists alike will tell you that a diet should be a way of life based on meeting your body's nutritional needs, not an isolated and ever-changing event based on the fad of the month. A look around your favorite bookstore might cause you to wonder if anyone's listening, though. It seems that there's a special diet for every conceivable circumstance. Won't just one diet do?

## The Good, the Bad ... the Diets

Most diets focus on certain foods or food groups, either to emphasize them or exclude them. Popular diets in recent years have encouraged people to eat all the protein they want but cut out carbohydrates, to eat as much pasta as they want but no meat, to drink only special preparations, and to eat only certain foods such as cabbage or rice. Most of these diets target weight loss. Although you might lose weight in the short term, your body will eventually rebel to restore its natural balance.

Doctors and nutritionists will tell you that the only good diet (and be sure to consult a licensed health professional before beginning any new diet regimen) is one that delivers the nutrients that your body needs. Fruits and vegetables dominate such a diet, as the USDA Food Guide Pyramid (see Chapter 13) shows, accompanied by whole grains and cereals, protein, and low-fat dairy products. Essential in smaller quantities are meats, processed baked goods, and sugars that deliver fats, proteins, and carbohydrates.

## Healthy Weight Control: Forget Deprivation and Get Off the Scale!

Does this mean that you shouldn't diet? In the sense that most women think of it—depriving yourself of calories or certain foods—dieting is counterproductive. Your body and your mind will soon revolt, sending you back to your old ways or even into a cycle of splurging on those formerly forbidden goodies. If you need to lose weight, be sensible. You didn't develop your tastes for favorite foods overnight, and you won't miraculously wake up tomorrow morning craving apples instead of donuts. Make small changes over time. These are easier to sustain and help you permanently change your tastes as well as your eating habits.

If you've always viewed the scale as your enemy, consider your hostility validated. Weight fluctuates not only from day to day, but also throughout the day, depending how much you're eating, drinking, urinating, and sweating. Many women experience weight swings with their menstrual cycles that can add up to several pounds. So get off the scale! If you must weigh yourself (for example, to monitor improvements in your BMI), do it just once a week—on the same day, at the same time, in the same place, and on the same scale. All the rest of the time, focus on what you're doing to improve your health—eating nutritiously, exercising regularly, and getting enough sleep at night. Before long, you won't need a scale to measure your progress.

Weight loss is a short-term goal. You've reached a point in your life at which short-term goals really don't meet your needs anymore (they probably didn't before, either, but let bygones be bygones). This is your opportunity to make a long-term investment in the future of your health. If weight loss is a piece of that goal, great! But keep it at that—just a piece. Focus instead on changing your lifestyle to support the person that you want to be.

> **Embracing Change**
>
> It takes at least two weeks for your taste buds to adjust to new flavors and sensations, whether you're adding or removing foods from your diet. Make changes one at a time to allow this adjustment to take place.

## The Curse of the Extra 10 (or So) Pounds

Sorry, girlfriends, but body fat does become a challenge in midlife. Even if you've made healthy eating and regular exercise part of your lifestyle for decades, you may hit 50-ish and find—gasp!—flab and spread where once there was fit and trim. At menopause, your middle wants to thicken. Your changing hormones affect your body's fat distribution patterns and also the amount of calories that your body needs to fuel its functions.

To an extent, this is one of those changes that you have to accept. Notice that we said "to an extent," though—we don't mean that you have to sit around and watch the flab spread. By all means, continue your good health habits—they serve many purposes beyond supporting your shape. And if you're overweight, do what you can to lose those extra pounds. But be aware that you won't again have the same body that you had when you were 20.

The good news is that you can have a body that's even healthier than the one you had when you were 20. You're not only older, but also wiser. The truth is, you know more about your body and what it needs than you've known at any other stage of your life. Menopause is a time for getting in touch with your knowledge and using your wisdom to shape your future. After all, what did you know about what lay ahead in your life when you were 20? Your resilient and forgiving body carried you through many experiences without you even noticing its gallant efforts. But you've learned a thing or two along the way, and now it's time for you to guide your body into the next stage of its (and your) future by making health-conscious choices.

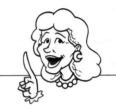

# Cultivating Healthy Eating Habits

Eating for your health doesn't mean giving up all the foods you've come to savor. It might mean finding new ways to prepare your favorites, or finding new taste sensations to balance your cravings and preferences. Taste is a learned thing. You're not born liking and disliking certain foods. You develop your likes and dislikes over time, sometimes more because of someone else's tastes than your own. If you have a favorite food that scores pretty low on the nutrition scale, go ahead and enjoy it once in a while. Just don't make it a dietary staple. You might be surprised to discover that, over time, you lose your taste for it.

## Whole or Refined: Does It Matter?

Nutritionists recommend whole grains over refined grains hands down. Whole grains and the products made with them retain significantly more nutrients than their refined counterparts (think about those big bakery donuts or packaged cookies …). White flour and white rice are common refined grains in Western diets. Look on the shelves of your local organic or health food grocer, and you'll see the wide variety of whole grains, whole-grain flours, whole-grain breads, and other food products just waiting for your discovery. It's a healthy diet change that's simpler to make than you might believe. And many good cookbooks give recipes for whole-grain ingredients, as well as how to substitute them in recipes that originally called for refined grains. Try whole grains; it will really make a difference. Read food labels in your traditional grocery store carefully and opt for products prepared with whole grains whenever such alternatives are available.

## Stay Close to the Source

Fresh is best when it comes to fruits and vegetables. Produce picked at the peak of ripeness contains the highest levels of natural nutrients. Because plants draw their nutrients from the soil, their supply ends with the harvest, and the nutrients they contain will gradually lose potency. If you can or want to grow your own garden, great. Gardening gives you both fresh produce and good exercise. It's also a wonderful way to relieve stress. But if you can't or don't want to plant your own vegetables, herbs, and fruits, that's fine, too. With modern transportation and storage procedures, you can buy fresh produce year-round.

Many people like to buy *organically grown* produce. In most cases, there is little nutritional difference between such produce and conventional produce. However, organically grown fruits and vegetables may have fuller flavor and texture because they're picked at peak ripeness and have a shorter selling period before they begin to wilt. They also don't have any chemical residues that could interfere with taste or present problems for people with sensitivities or allergies to certain chemicals.

**Wise Up**

Produce that is **organically grown** is planted, cultivated, harvested, and stored without any chemical additives such as fertilizers, insecticides, herbicides, and preservatives.

## Healthy Portions

It would be nice if you knew that a serving was a serving was a serving, no matter what you were eating. Unfortunately, portion sizes vary among foods and sometimes among manufacturers. Labels sometimes claim ridiculous portion sizes in an effort to keep servings within certain boundaries, such as fat content or calorie count. When was the last time you bought a small bag of pretzels or a bottle of juice and consumed just half? As often as not, how much we eat contributes more to excess intake than what we eat.

Get in the habit of reading labels. The portion size for most servings of meat and fish, for example, is 3 ounces, a piece roughly the size of a deck of cards. If you eat more than that, you're eating more than one serving. This not necessarily a problem, as long as you're aware of the nutritional consequences. And for some foods, it really doesn't matter. You can eat nearly as many servings of fruits and vegetables as you want, for example, as long as you don't exclude other necessary foods.

## Troublesome Favorites: Caffeine, Cola, and Chocolate

Ah, the three Cs: caffeine, cola, and chocolate. Can you live without them? The good news is, you don't have to remove them entirely from your diet. You do want to enjoy them with discretion, however. Caffeine is both a stimulant and a diuretic: It gets you wired and then sends you trotting off to the bathroom. Too much can leave you feeling frazzled and irritable, just what you need when your hormones are already sending you into the same territory. Chocolate and colas both contain caffeine, which can quickly add up to a good (or bad) case of the jitters.

Colas present a more serious hazard. The phosphoric acid that makes colas (and root beers) what they are acts like a bank robber when it gets into your body, holding up the Bank of Bone to steal calcium. In more technical terms, phosphoric acid binds with calcium, drawing it from your bones. Instead of putting the calcium to good use elsewhere in your body, however, this bonding process traps the calcium, which eventually is excreted in your urine. When you have precious little calcium to spare, drinking colas can speed you into osteoporosis before you know what's happened. Noncola sodas, although still empty calories, don't contain phosphoric acid.

It's not just your imagination: You really do feel better when you eat chocolate (especially *good* chocolate). Chocolate contains various chemicals that act on the neurotransmitters in your brain, stimulating the release of natural substances that improve your mood and soothe your stress. And the stearic acid in dark chocolate may be good for your heart, according to recent studies, by helping to lower your blood cholesterol levels. But in the end, chocolate, too, fills you with empty calories that quickly convert to you-know-what. Go ahead, indulge yourself with an occasional chocolate treat. Just don't make chocolate one of your major food groups.

# Foods for a Healthy Menopause

So what should you eat for a healthy menopause? First, follow the general nutritional guidelines for balance and moderation in your diet. Choose foods that are low in fat (especially saturated fat) and cholesterol. Eat lots of fruits and vegetables—the fresher, the better. Go for whole grains as much as possible, to get maximum nutritional value as well as an adequate level of dietary fiber. And eat foods that contain phytoestrogens to help relieve the discomforts of menopause.

## Back to Soy

So many health benefits can be had from soy, as we discussed in Chapter 19, "Soy, Herbs, and Other Botanicals: Nature's Menopause Miracles," that it would be a serious omission to exclude it from your diet. On the menopause front, soy reduces hot flashes and vaginal dryness, eases mood swings, and may increase bone density to help prevent osteoporosis. On the general health side, soy lowers blood cholesterol levels, helps prevent hormone-driven cancers, and is an excellent low-fat substitute for meat. And there are just about as many ways to add it to your diet! If you don't like soy-based foods, add powdered soy isoflavones to casseroles, sauces, and fruit smoothies.

## Flaxseed Oil, Fish, and Omega-3

Flaxseed oil has been around for thousands of years. Its main ingredients are a trio of essential fatty acids: stearic, linoleic, and alpha linoleic. These substances are called *essential* because your body needs them but can't make them itself, so it must get them through the foods you eat. These particular ones, called omega-3 fatty acids, are important during menopause because they suppress hormones called prostaglandins that cause uterine cramping (and are also linked to migraine headaches). Certain fish—salmon, tuna, mackerel, anchovies, sardines, and herring—are good sources of omega-3 fatty acids, which also help prevent heart disease.

# Vitamins and Minerals for Menopause

Whenever your body is going through a transition, it needs the support of additional vitamins and minerals. Some vitamins and minerals have particular benefits during the menopause transition. You can often supply your body with these needed nutrients through food choices. Many women find it more convenient and consistent to take supplements.

## Vitamin C and Citrus Bioflavonoids

Vitamin C is an important *antioxidant* that appears to have cancer-fighting capabilities. It helps to strengthen your immune system, replenishes collagen (a form of connective tissue) in your body, keeps bacteria levels low in your urinary tract, and maintains efficient cell function. Vitamin C also has mild estrogenic effects, stimulating your adrenal glands and helping to reduce vaginal dryness.

Foods that are good sources of vitamin C include oranges, grapefruit, tomatoes, broccoli, squash, melon, strawberries, and green, leafy vegetables, such as spinach and bok choy. Vitamin C is also available in supplement form, most commonly as a pill that you swallow or a tablet you chew. Natural sources of citrus bioflavonoids include the white, fleshy inner peel of citrus fruits. Citrus bioflavonoids are also available in capsules.

**Wise Up**

An **antioxidant** is a substance that binds with the byproducts of metabolism (called free radicals) to keep them from becoming poisons within your body. Scientists believe that free radicals play a role in the development of cancer.

## Calcium and Vitamin D

Calcium and vitamin D are critical during and beyond menopause to keep your bones healthy and strong to prevent osteoporosis. As you enter your 50s and 60s, your body's ability to extract calcium from the foods you eat becomes less efficient. So, you have to eat more to get less. The ability of your body to make new bone also diminishes, making it important to retain and strengthen the bone tissue that you already have. Doctors recommend that most women begin taking calcium supplements as they enter menopause and continue them for the rest of their lives.

Although calcium gets the most attention, it can't do its job without vitamin D. Vitamin D makes it possible for your body to use calcium and phosphorous, another mineral important to bone development. A little bit of vitamin D goes a long way, though. It's a fat-soluble vitamin, meaning that your body stores extra amounts in fat tissue throughout your body. Exceeding the recommended dose can allow vitamin D to accumulate to harmful levels.

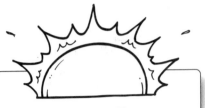

Most dairy products, processed orange juice, and many cereals are fortified with calcium and vitamin D. These substances are also available in numerous forms as supplements. Foods that are high in calcium include dairy products (go for the low-fat varieties), legumes, canned fish (with bones), rhubarb, spinach, bok choy, and cooked sea vegetables including hijiki, wakame, agar-agar, and kelp.

## Beta Carotene and Vitamin A

Beta carotene and vitamin A help keep your skin healthy and your mucous membranes moist. This reduces vaginal dryness and offsets the effects of reduced collagen (a consequence of low estrogen levels). Beta carotene is an antioxidant that converts into vitamin A in your body. Vitamin A is a fat-soluble vitamin best known for its effects in keeping your eyes and vision healthy. Food sources of beta carotene and vitamin A include dark green, leafy vegetables (such as spinach); cod liver oil; and egg yolks. Use supplements of these substances with care, and don't exceed the recommended daily doses. Vitamin A can accumulate to harmful levels because your body stores excess amounts.

# Get Moving: The Role of Exercise

There's so much to say about the benefits of exercise that we've dedicated an entire chapter to it later in this book (see Chapter 25, "Exercise: Menopause Magic"). But we have to say here that exercise is an essential aspect of a nutritious lifestyle. Exercise motivates your metabolism, getting your cells to function at their optimal levels. Exercise improves cell sensitivity to insulin, allowing body tissues to use glucose (sugar) efficiently. And exercise makes you feel better, which is never a bad thing!

### The Least You Need to Know

➤ You learned your tastes in food, and you can learn new tastes.

➤ Being overweight presents added health risks for 60 percent of Americans.

➤ Diets that deprive seldom achieve the lifelong changes necessary for healthy choices in eating.

➤ Focus on improving your health rather than losing weight, and you'll accomplish both.

➤ Vitamins and minerals can help your body travel more smoothly through menopause.

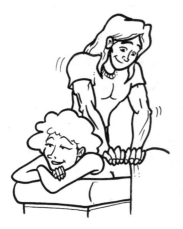

# Acupuncture, Biofeedback, Massage, and More

No matter what choices you make about HRT and hormone support, you can use many nonmedical techniques to navigate your menopause journey and find relief from the discomforts that you may encounter along the way. It'll probably take some exploring and experimentation to find out what various alternatives can do for you and whether they work better alone or in combination with others. But the process will give you a deeper and more comprehensive understanding of the most important person in your life: you.

Some approaches to smoothing the path, such as acupuncture, are thousands of years old. Others, like biofeedback, are decidedly modern. Many approaches seek to blend the best of old and new to provide a truly integrative experience.

## Integrating Alternatives into Menopause Care

Alternatives are what doctors often call adjunct therapies—you use them in addition to other treatments as a secondary line of symptom management. Beyond the boundaries of this clinical view, many alternative methods support you in a holistic way.

They look at individual discomforts in terms of how they affect the balance of your entire being—body, mind, and spirit—and then attempt to restore that balance. To integrate is to make the parts into a whole.

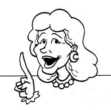

## Learning What's Available During Menopause

Many women are surprised to learn that treatments such as acupuncture, chiropractic, and massage therapies can provide relief during menopause. These approaches are outside the typical realm of allopathic medicine, or at least beyond the scope of the conventional allopathic physician. If you've chosen a regular doctor who supports integrative therapies, ask about alternatives that can complement or supplement any conventional treatment you're taking.

One of the best ways to find out what's working for other women going through menopause is to ask them. Among your friends and co-workers are women all along the continuum of, shall we say, maturity. Even if chatting about menopause isn't part of your routine conversations, most women are eager to share their experiences, both good and bad. And most of us are relieved to discover that we're not the only ones having bewildering experiences, such as forgetfulness or difficulty concentrating, that don't seem to fit the preconceptions that we might have about menopause. It's nice to share these concerns, as well as the solutions.

## Are Complementary Therapies Right for You?

Just as with HRT or herbal remedies, there's no universal "right" therapy for managing your menopause discomforts. What works for you depends on your unique circumstances and on what other therapies you're using. It's important to think of these alternatives as complementary—they can support and enhance other treatments. You might not get much relief from acupuncture, or you might find that your hot flashes seem to have vanished. You'll need to explore the various options to see what benefits they provide for you.

As with all healthcare choices, make these after verifying credentials. Some practitioners are subject to state regulations or licensing requirements, while others are not. A qualified practitioner should be pleased to show you evidence of his or her training and experience, and to provide references (check at least two or three). If you encounter reluctance, move on. If complementary therapies are new territory for you, start your quest by seeking recommendations from friends, co-workers, or neighbors.

Ask your regular doctor, your primary care physician, too. Doctors who support integrative care often have contacts among practitioners that they know to be reputable and qualified.

# Acupuncture: Ancient Tradition, Modern Therapy

Acupuncture is a mainstay of traditional Chinese medicine (TCM). This ancient therapy originated in China at least 5,000 years ago (and is possibly even older, but written records don't go back far enough). Artifacts recovered from archeological sites in parts of China included bone fragments sharpened into needles. Although the needles are now made of stainless steel no thicker than a few strands of hair, in most other respects the practice of acupuncture has remained virtually unchanged through the centuries.

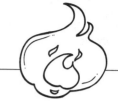

**Hot Flash!**

We've said this before, but it's important enough to bear repeating: Always check with your primary care physician before starting any new therapies. Your doctor doesn't have to agree with your decisions, but he or she needs to know what else is happening in your life that could affect your health.

Acupuncture is relatively new in the West. Travelers to the Far East in the 1800s came back from their adventures with stories of miraculous cures, witnessed or experienced, in which healers ceremoniously inserted needles into parts of the body seemingly not related to the sufferer's pain. However, these amazing stories remained the domain of travel lore until the 1970s, when a journalist traveling in China had his appendix removed. That's not a remarkable event by most standards—except that the only anesthesia his surgeons used was acupuncture. He wrote of his experiences, and the world awakened to a new—actually, old—form of therapy.

## Body, Mind, and Spirit Unified

In the Eastern view, body, mind, and spirit link to form the unified system that is your existence. Although body, mind, and spirit have distinctive roles and functions, they exist in balance with each other. Whatever affects one also affects the others. The life energy *chi* nourishes and connects all three dimensions. Chi's two components, *yin* and *yang,* coexist as a pair. When your yin and yang energies are balanced, you enjoy harmony and health. When your yin and yang energies become imbalanced—that is, when one dominates the other—you experience discomforts and illnesses. Healing is the process of restoring balance.

*The ancient symbol for the balance of yin and yang energies.*

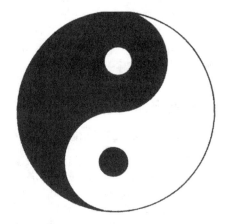

## Wise Up

**Chi** is the life energy that supports your existence. Its two components are the opposites yin and yang. **Yin** represents the cool, dark, moist, passive, and feminine. **Yang** represents the warm, light, dry, active, and masculine.

# Meridians: The Highways of Your Body's Energy Network

Chi flows through unseen channels in your body called *meridians*. There are 12 primary and 8 secondary meridians. In terms of location, meridians roughly follow your body's network of nerves. (However, there is no connection between the two systems.) The 12 primary meridians exist as pairs that channel chi through your organ systems. Two of the secondary meridians are paired, while the other four are not. The secondary meridians circulate chi to your emotional, psychological, and spiritual dimensions. Yin chi flows along the central, or medial, meridians and moves from outside to inside. Yang chi flows along the side, or lateral, meridians and moves from inside to outside.

When chi can flow through the meridians without blockage or obstruction, it remains in balance and your existence is one of health. When an obstruction blocks a meridian, it disrupts the flow of yin or yang, creating an imbalance of chi and a situation of "unhealth." Obstructions can be physical, emotional, or spiritual, and can be large or small. Large obstructions are associated with major health disturbances, while small obstructions are associated with minor health disturbances.

## Unblocking the Flow

Acupuncture attempts to unblock obstructed meridians to restore the balance of chi (and your wellness). It does so by creating interruptions of its own. These might dislodge the obstruction, or redirect the flow of chi around it. There are nearly 2,000 acupuncture points along your meridians, and there isn't always a physical relationship between your discomforts and the acupuncture points that influence them. The acupuncturist inserts tiny needles into the points that correlate to your symptoms or discomforts. The acupuncturist might activate (rotate, pluck, scrape, or vibrate) inserted needles to produce specific effects. This, too, is painless—and also deeply relaxing for many people.

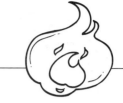

**Hot Flash!**

Your acupuncturist should use sterile, disposable needles to prevent the spread of infectious diseases such as hepatitis and AIDS. This is a legal requirement in most states in the United States and is the standard of practice nearly everywhere.

## Painless Needles (Really!)

No, it's not an oxymoron. If injections give you the heebie-jeebies, you can relax. In the hands of a skilled acupuncturist, acupuncture needles are painless. (You might feel a slight pressure or tingling, which acupuncturists call *deqi*, but nothing that hurts.) The needles are so fine, in fact, that four of them can fit inside a typical hypodermic needle used for giving injections.

If you just can't face the thought of needles of any size, consider acupressure or acumassage instead. In acupressure, the acupuncturist applies fingertip pressure (or sometimes an instrument made for this purpose) to the acupuncture point instead of inserting a needle. In acumassage, the acupuncturist massages along the meridian to stimulate the entire energy channel.

## Westernized Acupuncture: Tradition Meets Technology

It's hard for Westerners to leave well enough alone. We're always looking for ways to make old methods better. Acupuncture is no exception. Some acupuncturists blend modern technology with their ancient craft, using sound waves (sonopuncture) or mild electrical stimulation (percutaneous electrical stimulation, or PENS) to enhance the effects. There's also a trend among Western acupuncturists to view acupuncture (especially when enhanced by technology) as a therapy that stimulates your body's electrochemical balance rather than your chi balance. One theory supporting this view is that the inserted needles stimulate your body to release endorphins, which relieve pain and create a sense of mild euphoria or well-being. In fact, some therapies used to relieve chronic pain (such as transcutaneous electrical nerve stimulation, or TENS) use a form of electrostimulation that targets nerves just below the surface of the skin.

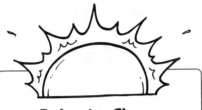

### Embracing Change

Whether your view of acupuncture is traditional and Eastern or modern and Western, one thing remains the same: Acupuncture does stimulate your body's healing mechanisms to bring you relief.

## *Choosing a Qualified Acupuncturist*

About 15,000 acupuncturists are licensed to practice in the United States, and about 4,000 of them are physicians with specialized training in acupuncture. Although there are various training programs for doctors, most combine at least 200 hours of classroom work and supervised practice. Because doctors already have extensive training in anatomy and physiology (the components of the human body and how they function), acupuncture training for doctors generally focuses on teaching acupuncture philosophies and methods.

TCM practitioners first receive comprehensive training in subjects such as anatomy and physiology, as well as diagnostics and other therapies such as herbals and medicinals. This intense training typically takes two to five years. Traditionally trained TCM practitioners learn the art of acupuncture from medical texts that have been in use for more than 2,000 years. A TCM practitioner then practices under the close supervision of an experienced TCM practitioner for another few years.

Not all states in the United States, and countries in the world, require these levels of education and experience, however. It's important for you to determine what training your acupuncturist has received. The best way to find out is to ask, and then check references. If in doubt, try someone else. You should feel comfortable with your acupuncturist's knowledge, skill, and interest in your health and needs. Acupuncture is helpful for relieving a variety of menopause discomforts, most notably hot flashes and abdominal aches.

# Biofeedback: Sending Messages to Yourself

Biofeedback is a technique of training your mind and your body to work together to achieve specific results. Some methods use small machines to measure and report particular body functions such as heart rate (pulse) and breathing rate. This is helpful when you're using biofeedback to relieve stress. Some people can use biofeedback to alter their pain responses, especially with migraine headaches and problems such as chronic back pain.

The use of biofeedback for hot flashes is based on our ability to regulate the thermostat of the individual. When vasodilalion occurs, there is a drop in skin resistance, which allows electrical impulses to pass on the skin's surface. By using this skin change as it is measured on the biofeedback equipment, the practitioner and woman use techniques such as breathing, relaxation, and self-talk to interrupt and alter the pattern of these changes. The effect is to reduce (and, with practice, hopefully eliminate) the hot flashes.

Biofeedback can be a useful tool for other menopause discomforts as well, including mood swings, headaches, stress, and PMS. It takes time and training to develop biofeedback skills. Ask your doctor to refer you to a reputable clinic or program so that you can learn the basic techniques.

# The Healing Power of Human Touch

We know the power of human touch from the moment of birth, when mother and child make first contact. Touch has the ability to soothe, comfort, and assure. It makes us feel loved and secure. In a therapeutic context, touch also can heal. It can restore blood flow, improve flexibility, and relieve aches and soreness. Many hospitals now offer healing touch to patients before and after surgery, to improve self-healing, lessen the effects of anesthesia, and reduce pain. Healing touch can help with PMS-like abdominal aches and cramps, hot flashes, headaches, and other menopause discomforts.

## Hands-On Healing: The Wide World of Massage

Nearly everyone enjoys a relaxing backrub. It takes your mind off whatever's bothering you, at least for a few minutes. It's like a good hug, only longer. But massage can do more than make you feel good. Therapeutic massage can improve circulation, helping to relieve discomforts such as fluid retention and PMS-like symptoms that often arise during menopause. Therapeutic massage stimulates your body to release endorphins, its natural "feel-good" substances, to take the edge off stress or mild depression. There are many kinds of therapeutic massage—here are some of the most common:

➤ **Shiatsu** is a form of Japanese massage that incorporates the principles of acupuncture to rebalance chi. The massage therapist uses fingers, palms, elbows, and even feet and knees to stimulate and apply pressure to acupuncture points. *Shiatsu* means "finger pressure."

➤ **Swedish massage** features various movements, from long strokes to focused kneading. Especially popular in health clubs and spas in the United States, Swedish massage is very relaxing and great for stress relief.

➤ **QiGong** is a form of massage in which the practitioner uses gentle touch to stimulate acupuncture points.

➤ **Tuina** is an ancient Chinese massage technique that combines massage and manipulation to release blockages from your meridians and restore the free flow of chi.

## Hands-Off Healing: Reiki

Sometimes the touch makes very little contact. *Reiki* is a Japanese healing method that calls on the practitioner to use her hands to focus the healing power of energy. The practitioner might gently touch your forehead for headaches, for example, or hold her hands over your lower abdomen (over the ovaries) for hot flashes. The practitioner concentrates on drawing energy through her hands and onto you, focusing and transferring its healing powers. This rebalances the flow of your chi.

Although Western cultures view Reiki with skepticism, the technique is widely respected and practiced in many other parts of the world. Reiki sessions can last an hour or so and generally leave you feeling profoundly relaxed and at peace. At the very least, this reduces stress and increases your sense of calm and well-being, which has numerous benefits for you during menopause discomforts and for your health in general.

**Wise Up**

**Reiki** is a Japanese healing method in which the practitioner uses her hands to focus energy over afflicted body parts. In translation, *reiki* means "universal vital force."

## Chiropractic: Removing Spinal Energy Blockages

The word *chiropractic* means "work of the hand." Chiropractors use their hands to adjust and manipulate your spine to restore its alignment. Even if it's not your back that's bothering you, you might find relief from menopause as seemingly unrelated to your back as hot flashes, fluid retention, and PMS-like symptoms. Although we think of chiropractic care as mainly focused on back health, chiropractic adjustments can function in much the same way as acupuncture and massage. From the Eastern perspective, chiropractic removes obstructions in the meridians (particularly those near the spine) and restores the balance and flow of chi. From the Western perspective, chiropractic relieves muscle tension and tightness to improve circulation to muscles and nerves.

Choose a chiropractor as you would select any healthcare practitioner. All states in the United States require chiropractors to be licensed, and most also seek certification in the states in which they practice. Ask for, and verify, the chiropractor's credentials and references. Your chiropractor should explain treatment options and recommendations in terms that you understand and should work with you to coordinate complementary therapies with any allopathic treatments that you're also taking.

## More Alternative Techniques to Try

A number of techniques exist to help you get in touch with the connections between your mind and your body. Most are easy to learn, and you can do them nearly anywhere, making them ideal for thwarting hot flashes and other discomforts in your living room, in your office, or even in a movie theater (if you don't mind missing a few minutes of the film). We discuss some of the Eastern methods, such as yoga, meditation, and tai chi, in Chapter 24, "Channeling the Energy Power of Menopause."

## Therapeutic Relaxation Methods

Stress intensifies many menopause discomforts, including sleep difficulties, problems with memory and concentration, mood swings and irritability, and even hot flashes. Methods such as deep breathing and conscious (progressive) muscle relaxation help you focus your mind to calm your body. You can do them separately or in combination to restore balance and give you a sense of tranquility.

> ➤ **Deep breathing**. These techniques are the foundation of many Eastern mind-body activities such as meditation and yoga. One simple technique is to stand with your feet comfortably apart and your hands at your sides. Close your eyes. Breathe in, slowly and deeply. Imagine that you can feel and see your breath drawing up from the soles of your feet, through your body, and out the top of your head. Hold the breath in your lungs, and feel its life-giving oxygen diffuse into your body. Breathe out, again slowly and deeply, and visualize your breath transporting the tension out of your body. Repeat six or seven times, until you feel calm and relaxed.

> ➤ Conscious (**progressive) muscle relaxation**. Sit or lie down with your body in an open position (no crossed arms or legs). Close your eyes. Choose a muscle that feels particularly tense. Focus on it. See it, feel it, and listen to what it would be telling you if it could speak. Concentrate on easing the tension from this muscle. Feel and see the muscle become relaxed and at rest. Move your attention to another muscle, and follow the same steps. At first it might take a while for your mind to connect with your body in this way, especially if you're accustomed to viewing your mind and body as separate entities. With practice, however, you can consciously relax your entire body in about 10 minutes.

## Visualization

Visualization is a mind-body activity that allows you to show your body, by using your mind, how you want it to feel. People who are proficient at this technique can often effectively halt hot flashes, headaches, and other discomforts even as they're

---

### Embracing Change

Chiropractors receive comprehensive training in both conventional and alternative therapies. A chiropractor might suggest breathing techniques to relieve stress, nutritional therapy to meet your body's nutritional needs, and meditation or biofeedback to empower your body's natural healing resources.

occurring. When you feel one of these signs coming on, stop what you're doing and focus your attention on it. Envision your emerging headache, for example, and then envision erasing it. Erase in circular motions, working from the center to the outsides. Then envision releasing the last wisp of discomfort with a slow, deep breath out. You can also use visualization in a preventive way by taking a few minutes throughout your day to sit calmly, eyes closed, and envision the state of your body as you want it to be: healthy, relaxed, and at peace with the changes taking place within it.

### The Least You Need to Know

➤ Most complementary (or alternative) therapies view your body as a unified system in which your body, mind, and spirit have equally important roles in your health and well-being.

➤ Complementary therapies are intended to support and enhance conventional therapies, not to replace them.

➤ Friends, neighbors, and your doctor are often your best sources for locating qualified, reputable practitioners of complementary therapies.

➤ Always check credentials and references. If you don't feel comfortable with a particular practitioner for any reason (or even no apparent reason), find someone else.

➤ There are many techniques for relaxation and healing that you can do yourself, no matter where you are.

# Part 6

# Self-Care While You're Going Through Menopause

*Your menopause experience is unique. But that's no reason to keep it to yourself. Menopause is no longer a journey that you must suffer in silence. Like other life passages, there are joys and tears, pains and reliefs, embarrassments and humor. How much more these experiences can connect you with the cycle of womanhood when you share them with other women who are on, or have completed, their menopause journeys!*

*The chapters in this part take a look at ways to draw strength from the vital energy that abounds when women share their experiences.*

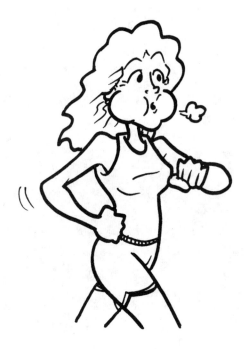

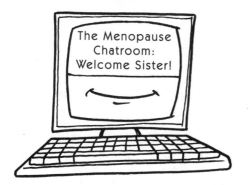

# Chapter 22

# This Is Not Your Mother's Menopause

> ## In This Chapter
>
> ➤ The value of shared experiences
>
> ➤ Using journaling to bring your dreams closer to reality
>
> ➤ Our unrealistic expectations of perfection
>
> ➤ How to love yourself for who you are

Do you remember your mother's menopause? She probably didn't talk much about it, just as she didn't talk much about other "woman" things. In spite of its universal nature, the menopause club has long been rather secretive about its membership. You didn't know you'd joined until you belonged. It was one of those events, like childbirth, in which the less was said about it, the safer you were.

Well, that has all changed. Menopause, like childbirth, has become an experience for us to savor despite its pains and in celebration of its joys.

## The Silent Passage Is Not So Silent Anymore

Yours—ours—is the first generation to experience widespread openness around matters of womanhood. Turn to any daytime talk show, and you're likely to find a discussion of pregnancy, PMS, sexual dissatisfaction, and even menopause. It's a far cry from the secrecy and embarrassment that confronted our grandmothers and mothers, who may not even have talked to each other about such subjects. The silent passage is no more.

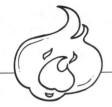

## Hot Flash!

Don't give out personal information in online chat groups. Not everyone who's in a chat room is who she (or he) appears to be. Most chat rooms allow or even encourage you to choose a screen name rather than using your real name. Don't let this anonymity lull you into a false sense of security about the information you share.

# From Support Groups to Cyber Chats and Beyond

Many communities have women's groups that gather for support on various topics related to menopause and midlife. Some are medical in orientation, addressing subjects such as HRT and hormone support therapies. Some focus on particular lifestyle issues—career crises, relationship challenges, or parenting pressures. Others might be spiritual or may list their meeting times and locations in local newspapers.

Online chat groups can put you in touch with people you'd otherwise never meet, across the country or even across the world. It's a great way to expand your knowledge and understanding of what this menopause transition means, in general and to specific women. You can share highlights, worries, symptoms, and remedies. You might discover that your unique problems are actually quite universal, or you might learn that a particular sign or symptom isn't typical and should be evaluated by your doctor.

The Internet has also broadened the base of available knowledge. Ten years ago you might have spent hours in a medical library researching the forms of HRT, but today you can gather information from the world's leading experts in a matter of minutes. It's entirely likely, in fact, that you'll end up knowing more than your doctor about alternatives and complementary therapies. Of course, it's important to have a healthy skepticism about information that you find on the World Wide Web. If something sounds too good to be true, it undoubtedly is. Gather information from reputable Web sites, and verify your research.

## Sharing What You Know

Women talk. We know it, our children know it, doctors know it, and men know it. Talking is one way in which we explore our experiences, as though the process of running the words through our thoughts lets us turn those experiences this way and that to get a closer look. Speaking puts structure to our thoughts, and hearing our own words come back to us gives them a new shape and dimension.

You have a private wealth of information about menopause, even if you feel bewildered and confused most of the time. Talking with other women lets you share your personal experiences as they relate to this universal journey. Your observations and knowledge then become your contributions to the collective wisdom of womanhood. Your words can provide the connections that other women are seeking and can link you with additional sources of information for yourself.

## *Journaling: Keeping Your Dream Book*

Often, all you have to do to get what you want is ask for it. But first you have to know what you want. In their book *The Aladdin Factor* (Berkeley Books, 1995), authors Jack Canfield and Mark Victor Hansen tell a story from their workshops. "We'll often ask people to make a list of what they want that they currently don't have," the authors write. "Invariably someone says more money. At that point we'll reach into our pockets, pull out a quarter, and give it to them." Of course, that's not what people have in mind.

What dreams and desires live in the back of your mind, hidden behind the demands and pressures that drive your everyday life? *Journaling* is one way to give shape to your ideas and thoughts, and even figure out how to make your dreams become realities in your life. As the example Canfield and Hansen use illustrates, you have to be specific. If you can't read your own mind, how can you expect other people to? Writing in your journal about what you want can help you clarify your desires, translating them into tangibles that are attainable.

Did you keep a diary when you were younger? This is a form of journaling in which you record events and circumstances that happen to you, and perhaps your thoughts about them. Some people start keeping a diary when they learn to write, and continue throughout their lives. Others begin journaling later in life, often in response to a life challenge or life-changing experience.

**Wise Up**

**Journaling** is the process of using writing to explore your thoughts and ideas.

Journaling is an opportunity for you to explore the depths of your feelings and aspirations without the pressures of sharing them with others. You can get comfortable with expressing your dreams and become familiar with them so that when the time comes to begin taking action to make them reality, you have no hesitation.

Journaling can be as formal or as casual as you want to make it. You can buy bound books with blank pages, or use loose-leaf notebook paper that you store in a three-ring binder or a folder. Most women find that the greatest benefit comes from journaling on a regular basis, usually daily. Set aside a time when you can write uninterrupted for 30 to 45 minutes. You can make this a ritual, using a special place and lighting a candle to help focus your mind and your energy.

# Our Mothers, Ourselves?

"When I grow up, I won't be anything like my mother, I swear!" It's the oath of many an adolescent perched on the brink of womanhood. But 20 or 30 years later comes the startling recognition: "I'm just like my mother!" Whether you view this as a

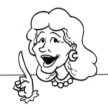

blessing or a curse is, of course, your unique and personal matter. But like it or not, the older you each become, the less that separates you. You may become friends—or not. You may become peers—or not. You may find that you have many interests and beliefs in common—or few.

All your life you've been moving along—maybe dragging your feet, maybe racing ahead—on the path that your mother's already traveling. Perhaps your mother has helped you on your journey, and you've helped her. Or maybe each of you has struggled through your separate challenges. Common experiences bond you in your solitary yet connected journeys as you come of age, gradually building the links that join you in the circle of womanhood.

You are not your mother, of course, despite the life transitions that put you both on common ground. Your experience of menopause is uniquely yours, no matter how universal aspects of it appear to be. But you do have more in common with your mother now than at any other time in your life. You've lived more years in each other's lives than not as your paths overlap during these years.

## Joining a Club That Has Your Mother as a Member

It's interesting (and somewhat disconcerting) to be a member of your mother's club, to see her as her woman friends see her and even as you see your woman friends. This is the woman who gave you life, kissed your cuts and scrapes, and held you in her lap long after you were too grown to fit there comfortably. Now she worries about breast cancer, wonders if she should be taking HRT, muses about sex, and contemplates whether to color her hair—your issues, too. And you might be a mother yourself, with daughters following you who will some day join the circle themselves.

## Admission to the Wise Woman Club Is Freeing

One of the most refreshing discoveries about midlife is that there's so much less for you to worry about. For most women at this stage of life, there are no decisions to consider about having children, developing a career, or impressing your peers. Your life has shape and definition. Even if you decide, at this crossroad, that you want to make changes, you have a framework in place that you can remodel. You don't have to build from scratch. In fact, there are many things that you don't *have* to do at all anymore, if you choose. There's something empowering, almost magical, about reaching this point in your life. It's exhilarating to decide to do things—or not—solely because they appeal to you, and to realize that you truly don't care what anyone else thinks. The realm of your world has vastly expanded, even as it appears to be narrowing.

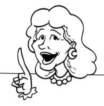

### Wise Woman's Wisdom

"People who have seen, felt, and incorporated their private truths during midlife no longer expect the impossible dream, nor do they have to protect an inflexible position. Having experimented with many techniques for facing problems and change, they will have modified many of the assumptions and illusions of youth. They are practiced. They know what works. They can make decisions with a welcome economy of action."

—Gail Sheehy

# A Notion of Perfection

Our Western culture is fixated on perfection. We want perfect bodies, perfect careers, perfect relationships, perfect children, and perfect houses with perfect yards in perfect neighborhoods. Although common sense and reality tell us that this kind of perfection is impossible, we nonetheless seek it, secretly believing that if only we try a little harder, perfection can be ours. It can't. Perfection is an unachievable ideal that exists only in the illusions that we create to support our belief that it should exist. Oh, do we love our illusions!

## *Perfect Bodies, Perfect Minds, Perfect Lives*

A book of guidance for women printed in the late 1800s quantified the ideal woman as 5 feet tall, with a waist no bigger around than 2 feet with a full bust and broad hips. Although few women have ever matched this ideal, it has been sought after for a century or longer. You can't say we haven't tried. Women have stuffed themselves into corsets, attached awkward and ungainly bustles to their backsides, and struggled to walk on high heels—all in pursuit of an hourglass figure. And when the dictates of the illusional ideal changed, so did women's efforts to match it.

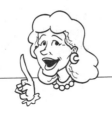

In the 1950s, the ideal woman—personified by the burgeoning specter of the supermodel—weighed in at 8 percent less than the average woman. She was buxom and robust—Betty Grable, Jane Mansfield, Marilyn Monroe. Thirty years later, the ideal had slimmed to a mere wisp of its former self—remember Twiggy? In the 1990s, the typical supermodel weighed in at 25 percent less than a woman of healthy weight. All around you, messages abound that support the illusion of perfection. Supermodel bodies strike supernatural computer-graphic–enhanced poses on the covers of magazines. Television relationships often glorify the melodramatic and stormy extremes of family and community experiences—but usually resolve themselves neatly in that perfect 30- or 60-minute episode. Isn't that movie kid oh so precocious and cute? Viewers are often left with TV solutions that are equally as far from everyday reality as the melodrama that sets the stories in motion. The disparities between media images of perfection and real life drive women to wonder what's wrong with their lives. Nothing. The ideal, as Hollywood and Madison Avenue present it to us, doesn't exist!

The *real* perfect body, experts agree, is one that's healthy and fit. Even in this era of concern about weight and appearance (at any given time, half of American women are dieting), what matters more are lifestyle habits that support good health. The only relationship that's ideal for you is the one that brings you joy and comfort. The dream job is the one that turns your dreams to reality, whether that's climbing the corporate ladder or doing what you can to make ends meet so that you can enjoy other aspects of your life such as travel, hobbies, or family. Kids, if they're a part of your life, will be kids—and they have their own missions. The genuine perfect life is the one that makes *you* happy. That's the ideal that matters—and that is, for most people, perfectly achievable.

## Even Martha Stewart Can't Escape Menopause

Menopause is a universal experience. If you're a woman, it's your destiny. No amount of fame, fortune, or foot-dragging will keep you from it. All women, in our flawed perfection, make this inevitable life passage. Go gracefully! (Not *perfectly* ....) Make the experience worthwhile. Let yourself enjoy the changes in your body and in your life. You'll emerge from your journey a little tired perhaps (this can be, after all, an arduous adventure), but amazingly stronger, more confident, and more competent than ever before.

## Craft and Artistry of the Ingenious Wise Woman

Even as we grow older, we become more creative. In part, our growing older forces this. If you can't outrun the competition (even if you're competing with only yourself), you have to learn how to outsmart it. Economy and efficiency become essential as you find new ways to manage the tasks and demands of your life.

Creativity often emerges in other ways at midlife, too. This could be the first time in your life that you let the artist in you come out. In part this is an element of reshuffling your priorities—at midlife, you realize that time is not unlimited. More importantly, you recognize that you're going to turn 50, 60, or 70 whether or not you take up pottery, playing the piano, or painting with watercolors. The artist within you finally feels free to venture out and stretch her talents.

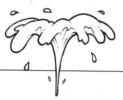

### Wellspring

True beauty, however you define it, never fades—think Sophia Loren or Elizabeth Taylor. Real beauty continues to glow bright and strong, even as it adapts and changes. What shows on the outside reflects an inner beauty that only deepens through time. Yes, your body is changing. You don't look the same as you did when you were 20, and you won't again. But inside you remain the same, no matter what your age (well, you do get a little wiser and a little bolder). Like fine wine, you become richer and fuller, but no less than what you've always been. Enjoy and appreciate this new you!

# For Now, the Inner Revolution

The changes that you see when you look in the mirror barely scratch the surface of what's taking place within you—not just within your body, but within your mind and your spirit as well. Menopause is a journey along life's path, a journey of exploration and examination as much as a trip through time. It's a time of spiritual growth as you try to figure out what you've accomplished on this mission that is your life, and what remains for you to complete. You may find yourself realigning the outward appearances of your life to reflect your core values. Others might view this process with alarm, questioning why you're changing so much. Yet in your mind, you're not changing at all—you're just becoming the person you've always been.

## *Gloria Steinem, Are You Listening?*

The generation of women now approaching menopause are children of the revolution. We fought for the right to be ourselves, to enjoy choices and lives free from artificial constraints imposed upon us by arbitrary, gender-oriented standards. We burned our bras and braved new worlds, upending the expectations that our mothers had for us (often to the accompaniment of their cheers). Now we stand at the edge of yet another transition, another border of challenges and expectations. Are we going quietly along the path just because the path is well-trodden? No way! Even as we embrace the endless cycle that draws us along, we're storming the gates. We want this stage of our lives to be just like the others—we want to take charge, to be in control. We've learned our lessons well. We didn't live our mothers' lives, and this isn't our mothers' menopause.

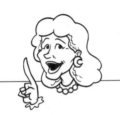

**Wise Woman's Wisdom**

*"Age is all imagination. Ignore years and they'll ignore you."*

—Ella Wheeler-Wilcox

## Mirror, Mirror ...

What do you see when you look at the face staring back at you from the mirror? (Go ahead, put on your glasses so that you can see it.) Do you wonder who that person is and how she got to where she is in her life? Do you admire her? It isn't always easy to see the changes that your body is experiencing, until that one day when you look in the mirror and there they are, facing you. A few lines around the eyes, a little droop under the chin, a sprinkling (or more) of gray hair. This is the face, the image, of life itself. You are woman, in all her incarnations. Take a closer look, and get to know that woman in the mirror—the beautiful reflected face of a life lived with vitality, a lovely face that has earned the beauty that comes with the confidence of experience that a young face, however eager, cannot match.

## Loving What It Means to Be You

This is your life, and this is your time. You have become who you are—and, odds are, it pleases you. You are coming into your own in ways that you never dreamed possible. It's a little scary—and a little exciting. For many women, it's also comforting. Finally, they can dispel pretensions and be themselves. The funny thing is, this is often more of a discovery for us than for the people in our lives who have always loved us for who we really are. Now it's time for us to do the same.

## The Least You Need to Know

➤ Sharing your menopause experiences with other women broadens your understanding of what's happening within you and what to expect as your journey continues.

➤ To get what you want from this journey and from life, often all you have to do is ask.

➤ Although women through all of time have traveled this same path, you don't have to walk in their footsteps. Make your journey your own by tuning in to your inner needs and changes.

➤ Love yourself for who you are.

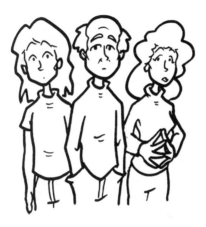

# Chapter 23

# Well-Meaning Family, Friends, and Co-Workers

### In This Chapter

➤ What menopause means to others in your life

➤ How to fulfill your need to nurture

➤ Remaining comfortable with your decision to stay child-free

➤ The career implications of being older

➤ The true value of friends

As much as your menopause journey is uniquely yours, there are others who are traveling your path with you—some willingly, some begrudgingly. Your experiences affect your family members nearly to the extent that they affect you. They're unsettled, too, that you're not yourself anymore (even if you feel that you're becoming more like the self that you really are). As much as you want to reassure them that you're the same old you, you're not sure of this yourself.

Being menopausal is a lot like being a middle child. You're not quite young, not quite old. (If you happen to be a middle child, you may know the feeling of "not quite" all too well.) You might even feel that you don't really fit anywhere at this point in your life. Although this might be disconcerting, it's not uncommon. This is the most significant transition in your life since puberty ushered you into adulthood 30 or 40 years ago. It's perfectly normal to feel a bit disoriented. Don't worry, you will get yourself back. It's just going to take a little time.

# When You Feel Like Yourself ... But You Don't

In the meantime, try to go with the flow. Pay attention to how you feel. Perhaps there are messages in your confusion and discomfort. For many women, midlife triggers a process of assessment and evaluation. Your sense of feeling lost and out of place could be telling you that it's time to make some long-overdue changes in your life. Rather than again rearranging the furniture, maybe you need to move to a house that's more like the dream home that you've always imagined calling yours. Instead of trudging off to yet another day at the office, take a "mental health day" to examine your reluctance to leave the house in the morning. Are you in a job that you don't like, or are there a few simple changes that you could make that would turn things around?

Once you tune into your feelings, you can often identify the underlying issues and concerns that are feeding them. Sometimes just the process of identification changes the way you feel. Other times, it leads you to the changes that you need—and want—to make.

# All in the Family

Because it can be difficult to convey your experiences and your feelings to those who can't physically and emotionally share them, you may not get the support and understanding that you need from your family. After all, what's the big deal about feeling flushed for a few minutes? You know, of course, that it's much more than a few minutes' worth of flushing. But try explaining that to someone who doesn't have ovaries ....

## Of Menopause and Men

Menopause is a mysterious and often frightening event for the men in your life to witness, especially the man who is your husband or partner. Your experiences may trigger his own worries about growing older. Some of his concerns are the same as yours—will you still find each other attractive, will you still want and enjoy sex, and will everything still stay the same? Well, of course, nothing ever really stays the same. It's just that you're not the person he thought he knew, and that's confusing for both of you.

Tell your partner what kind of support you want him to provide for you. Do you want him to listen without comment when you talk about menopause matters, or do you want him to offer his observations and insights? Should he tell you when he thinks you're being outrageous or unreasonable, or should he just humor you until the mood or situation passes? How do you want him to let you know when he's angry or upset with your feelings and behaviors? If the two of you already have a good foundation for communication in place in your relationship this transition in your life will be just a matter of minor adjustments and clarifications. If communication is like a narrow, one-way street in your relationship, where each of you struggles for passage, then you could be in for a rough and rocky ride. But you can emerge stronger and more solid in your relationship if you're both willing to give and take.

## Of Menopause and Being a Mother

You might be working through your feelings about lost fertility without even realizing that you're doing so, particularly if you have children who are now grown and are moving away from the nest. Even if you've also had a career all during the years you were raising kids, all that kid stuff occupied a great deal of your time, emotions, and thoughts. Now that it's all behind you, you might be wondering what you did with all that energy before you had kids—and what you're going to do with it now.

There are no universal answers. Some women transition smoothly from the child-oriented phase of their lives to other interests. Some women struggle to rediscover who they really are. Many women are somewhere in between. All of this is a normal and natural part of your transition. Take comfort in knowing that you will resettle on the other side. And draw on your support network—significant other, close friends, and other family members—to help you work through your feelings and concerns. Although we tend to view menopause as the end of fertility, it's also the beginning of new growth for you. Celebrate the menopause life passage as an opportunity to explore new challenges and nurture yourself, as you've nurtured others.

**Embracing Change**

If your need to nurture remains strong after your children leave home, consider volunteering with local community or service organizations that work with youth. From daycare centers to scout troops, there are abundant opportunities for you to share the lives of young people.

## Of Menopause and Being a Grandmother

Did you ever wish that you could enjoy your children when they were at their best, and not have to deal with them when they weren't? If you're a grandmother, your wish has come true! You can play with the kids for a while and then go home to a hot cup of tea, a good book, and absolute silence if you want it. Being a grandmother is like returning to mothering while leaving all the responsibilities behind.

It isn't easy for some women to adjust to the thought of being grandmothers. Part of this is a holdover from our own childhoods, when we looked upon our grandparents as ancient beings tottering on the edge of death. They weren't, of course. It's just that, as a child, your sense of relativity is a bit skewered. You're so very young, so anyone who's not looks so very old. With many women of your generation waiting until later in their lives to establish their families (or establishing new families with new partners), you could have grandchildren older than your best friend's children. As disconcerting as this might be, it's increasingly common. One thing for which you can be thankful, however, is that at least you won't have adolescence and menopause in your house at the same time!

## Amazon, Without the Dot.Com: Life Child-Free

Before it became known as the Internet's megabookstore, an Amazon was a mythical warrior-woman noted for her ability to remove a breast to make it easier to draw back her bow. (Those ancient Greeks had quite the imaginations!) Fierce and dedicated, these fabled fighters had a single mission: combat. And by most accounts, they excelled at it. But they did nothing else. They didn't marry or raise children. The Amazons were the original career women, putting aside everything for the sake of good battles.

Many women who entered adulthood in the 1960s and 1970s, and who are now entering menopause, made similar choices—not to do battle, although sometimes they felt like it (without arrows or removable breasts, of course), but to take on the wider world of opportunities traditionally reserved for men. Increasingly, women are running businesses, traveling, marrying later in life, and postponing or forestalling child-rearing. Many also have chosen to remain unmarried and child-free—and are not branded "spinsters" for their choice. Now at midlife, these women find that they have the freedom to explore new adventures and build securely on the base of experience they've built along the way.

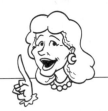

**Wise Woman's Wisdom**

"Time and trouble will tame an advanced young woman, but an advanced old woman is uncontrollable by any earthly force."

—Dorothy L. Sayers

If you are such a woman, you know that midlife marks the point of no return for some of the decisions that you made when you were younger. You're not likely to have children, for example. Even if you made a conscious choice to live child-free, it can still come as a shock to realize that your days of choosing on such matters are drawing to an end. And as gradually as your life's circumstances have evolved, it can still startle you to recognize that you're not 27 any more.

It can take a while to be okay with this. Yet for many women, there soon comes a sense of peace about the new status of midlife. Pregnancy is no longer a worry, nor is the pressure to "settle down and start a family." You can be who you are, and that's that! If you want to leave the country to spend three months abroad, start med school, or launch a dot.com company, there are few constraints holding you back. Women are no longer defined solely by their status of motherhood; you can embrace menopause as a celebration of who you have chosen to be.

# Menopause and the Working Woman

Experience is the classic dilemma for someone just entering the workplace. Without experience, you can't get a job. Without a job, you can't get experience. But what happens when you've been in the work force for long enough to acquire a good amount of experience? Does this work for or against you when you want to move up in your career? Much of the contemporary workplace structure still revolves around the model of the 1950s and 1960s, when men dominated the job environment and retirement was their ultimate objective. In this model, you worked your way as far up the ladder as you could go before you turned 65, and then you retired.

Experience was particularly an issue for working women of the time, who often were rejoining the workforce after taking 10 or 20 years off to raise families, or who were entering it for the first time. Starting their careers at age 35, 40, or older, they barely became established before it was time for a gold watch and a retirement party. Always behind those who had been in the work force all their adult lives, these women did not have time to develop the experience that they needed to move up in their careers before mandatory retirement cut short their efforts.

Then came the "gray revolution" of the 1970s. Inspired by the success of the woman's movement, older Americans pushed to end mandatory retirement, arguing that someone who wants to work into her 70s or even beyond shouldn't be prevented from doing so just because of age. The federal Age Discrimination in Employment Act (ADEA) of 1975 put the force of law behind this desire. Today, most people can work as long as they choose.

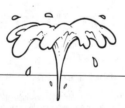

### Wellspring

In 1975, the U.S. Congress passed the Age Discrimination in Employment Act (ADEA). This federal law (known officially as 45 CFR Part 91) makes it illegal to hire, fire, or treat differently any individual between the ages of 40 and 70 solely on the basis of age. The ADEA applies to employers who have 20 or more employees. The U.S. Equal Employment Opportunity Commission (EEOC) investigates complaints about age discrimination and handles about 15,000 cases a year. In the year 2000, the American work force employed nearly four million workers age 65 and older.

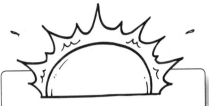

**Embracing Change**

If you think that you want to make a career change but aren't sure what you want to do, consider seeing a career consultant who can help you identify your strengths. Numerous tests can provide insights into your interests and inherent abilities. A career consultant can help you match your results to jobs and careers.

## Seasoned Executive Material or Over the Hill?

Does your boss see you as ripe for promotion or ready for retirement? It probably depends on whether you've stayed abreast of new developments in your field or profession—or persisted in doing things the same old way. Even as businesses appreciate the value that experienced employees bring to the work force, they recognize the need to cultivate a skill base that can carry them into the future, not tie them to the past. Younger workers arrive full of fresh ideas. They're eager to implement their innovations, to establish themselves as valued and respected employees. Companies, of course, welcome this "new blood," hoping that it will infuse the bottom line.

But innovative thinking is not the exclusive domain of the young. Older workers can be just as creative, and they have the added advantage of knowing what already does or doesn't work—and often why. Most employers would rather keep current workers than train new ones. The challenge is to be sure that your employer knows that you want to stay and that you are continuing to make vital contributions.

## Coping Strategies for the Workplace

When was the last time you learned something new about or for your job? If you can't remember, you could be in trouble. Sign up for classes and workshops, subscribe to (and read) professional publications, and listen to cafeteria conversations. Opportunities for learning are all around you. If you suddenly find yourself the office senior citizen, look for ways to make that your advantage. Let your expertise show. (Don't flaunt it—just let it speak for itself.) Be willing to mentor younger co-workers if they want your guidance and suggestions. (Don't push yourself on them as the resident expert—just be there.) It's not always easy, especially if you figured that by now you'd be enjoying the status of seniority. But it accomplishes the same goals that your younger co-workers are working toward: demonstrating that you are a valuable and vital member of the organization.

## Rebirthing Your Career: Creating Your Own Opportunities

Midlife is a time of career reassessment and change for many women. You might have worked in a particular job or field because that was where you started and other aspects of your life have taken priority until now. Perhaps what you really wanted to do wasn't feasible earlier in your life because you didn't have the education or the experience, or the job opportunities weren't there. And sometimes things just change—your interests, your needs, your circumstances.

By midlife, finances and families are often stabilized. The pressure to produce has eased, and you finally have a chance to look at other interests. It's a good time to go back to school, start your own business, or shift to work that you can do from home so that you can set your own hours. Or maybe you want to take a part-time job just to pay your bills, and spend the rest of your time pursuing hobbies or other interests. With the typical American now progressing through several careers (not just jobs) in a lifetime, it's never too late to try something new.

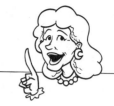

**Wise Woman's Wisdom**

"A friend doesn't go on a diet because you are fat. A friend never defends a husband who gets his wife an electric skillet for her birthday. A friend will tell you she saw your old boyfriend— and he's a priest."

—Erma Bombeck

# Friends Forever

Through the timeline of your life, you've developed various circles of friends—some in childhood, some at college, some at work, some in the places you live, and some who are the parents of your children's friends. And for much of your life, these circles tend to stay distinct from one another. You see work friends at work and neighborhood friends when you're doing yard work or attending community meetings. Visiting childhood friends is a great treat when you go back to your hometown or they come to your city. You might know the parents of your children's friends only by their first names, yet you feel that you know each other well through the intimate details that you learn about each other's lives through what the kids say.

Over time, you draw from these many circles to develop a small, inner ring of the friends who become the ones with whom you share your deepest secrets, from how much you really weigh to what you believe about life after death. Your bonds with the few women who make up this inner circle are often deep and intertwining, and the crises of your lives draw you even closer. By midlife, your relationships with your best friends have survived marriages, children being born, children moving away from home, divorces, and even deaths.

These friends form your support network. Those who have already experienced menopause can provide reassurance and comfort—not to mention living proof that you, too, will survive this grand yet challenging adventure. Those who are on their menopause journeys can share your worries and joys. And you can provide guidance and support for those who are still on the outside looking in.

# Can I Help You with Those Groceries, Ma'am?

Do you remember the first time someone called you "ma'am"? If it stopped you in your tracks, your reaction was not uncommon. (And if you wanted to throttle the "youngster," that's not uncommon, either.) It's a jolt to suddenly realize that not only are you older than many of the people who cross your path every day, but also that they perceive you as older. Just exactly when did you become "older"?

You've been drifting toward it for quite some time, of course, and if you stop to think for a minute, you probably don't really remember the very first time someone called you ma'am. What you do remember is the first time that someone did and you found it annoying rather than amusing. It's an odd turning point in life, to look around and see that everyone appears to be younger than you. This is becoming an illusion. Despite the youth orientation of our society, it's the numbers of people over age 50 that are growing most rapidly. And more people over age 50 are in the work force than ever before. It's entirely likely that the "youngster" offering to help you with your groceries is older than you! Smile, and enjoy your newfound status.

---

### The Least You Need to Know

➤ The changes that you're experiencing are just as confusing (and sometimes frightening) to family members and friends as they are to you.

➤ A strong communication foundation can keep your relationship floating high during this challenging time.

➤ Many women choose this time in their lives to start new careers or pursue different interests.

➤ Your inner circle of friends can provide a lifeline of support and encouragement for you.

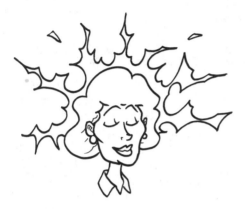

# Channeling the Energy Power of Menopause

There is a connectedness in this circle of transition that is your menopause journey. It's yet another round in the cycle of change, the cycle of life, the cycle that unites all women, through all time, in a common journey. Countless women before you have traveled, and countless women after you will travel, their separate paths on this same journey.

When we talk of menopause's power surges, it's often to make light of hot flashes. But there is a power beyond—beyond you and beyond each of us, a power that supports and connects us all in the endless cycle of time. Sound a little too much like the next sequel to *The Lion King?* Stay tuned!

## Your Body as a Map of the Universe

Eastern philosophies hold that your body is a vessel filled with life energy. It is a representation in miniature of a larger vessel of energy, the universe. Nothing happens within your body without altering the flow of energy in the universe, and all that happens in the universe affects the life energy that is your existence. The tides of energy thrust and tug at your body and your psyche (the mind-spirit that is your essential being), shifting and changing your physical, spiritual, and emotional dimensions. This constant movement carves the path of your life.

## Ancient Energy Systems for Vitality and Health

Ancient systems viewed health and illness as the balance and imbalance of energy. Although our modern perspective is that this typifies Eastern philosophies and practices, the premise is deeply rooted in Western medicine as well. The *doctrine of humors,* which linked vital body substances with particular sensory and environmental qualities, governed medical practice from the time of famed Greek physician Hippocrates (460–361 B.C.E.) until well into the Middle Ages. Greek scholars believed that the human body was a microcosm, or small representation, of the universe at large. The balance among blood, phlegm, yellow bile, and black bile correlated to the balance of air, water, fire, and earth as well as to the balance of hot, moist, cold, and dry.

**Wise Up**

The **doctrine of humors** was the ancient model of medicine based on the link between vital body fluids and the elements that those fluids represented. The doctrine of humors formed the core of Eastern and Western medical practices for thousands of years.

Imbalances altered physical and emotional health to produce conditions of disease and disturbance. The physician's mission was to identify the humor, element, or trait that was either excessive or lacking. Treatment aimed to restore balance, typically by reducing whatever was in excess. Bloodletting was a common therapy, accomplished through incisions into veins near the skin's surface (dangerous in a time when practitioners didn't understand the distinctions between veins and arteries). Restoring balance among the humors returned the body to harmony within itself as well as with the universe at large.

Ancient Eastern systems followed similar theories and approaches, although they were often more complex and more holistically focused. Ancient Eastern healers recognized chi, the life energy, as the thread that connected all life activities. Although Eastern healers also used methods such as bloodletting, their healing practices focused more on manipulating the flow of chi to regulate and restore the balance of the humors—and, correspondingly, the balance of health.

**Wise Up**

**Chakras** are centers of energy within your body. The word *chakra* means "wheel" in Sanskrit. **Nadis** are the unseen pathways that connect the chakras.

# East Meets West: Chakras and Your Spine

In Chapter 21, "Acupuncture, Biofeedback, Massage, and More," we talked about meridians, the unseen energy channels that circulate chi. Forming another dimension of your body's energy network are the *chakras*. Located along your spine, the seven chakras are like energy storage centers. Each chakra holds an accumulation of chi that correlates to a certain psychic or psychospiritual function. Connecting the chakras to one another are channels called *nadis*. The chakras also correspond to the body's major endocrine glands. Unlike meridians, which channel chi through your body, mind, and spirit without your conscious awareness, chakras must be activated to release the energy that they contain.

## The Seven Chakras

| Chakra | Location | Endocrine Gland | Energy | Color |
|---|---|---|---|---|
| First/Root | Base of spine | Ovaries/testes | Survival, kundalini | Red |
| Second/Spleen | Sexual organs | Pancreas | Sexuality, passion | Orange |
| Third/Solar | Solar plexus | Adrenals | Personal power, sense of self | Yellow |
| Fourth/Heart | Heart | Thymus | Love, compassion | Green |
| Fifth/Throat | Base of neck | Thyroid | Creativity, expression, communication | Blue |
| Sixth/Brow | Center of forehead ("third eye") | Pituitary | Clairvoyance, intuition, clarity of perception and understanding | Indigo |
| Seventh/Crown | Top of head | Pineal | Enlightenment, spirituality, connectedness to the universe | Violet |

# Synchronizing Chakra Energy During Menopause

As the previous chart shows, each chakra has a correlation to some aspect of menopause. The second chakra, for example, is located in your sexual organs and contains the energy of passion and sexuality. Correspondingly, your sexual organs contain and release the physical sensations of—you guessed it—passion and sexuality. The other chakras have similar correlations that link psychic and physical functions. Synchronizing or centering your chakras helps restore balance to this dimension of your being. Methods such as meditation and yoga, which strengthen the unity of your body and psyche (mind-spirit), are ways to achieve this harmony.

*The first chakra is at the base of the spine, and the seventh chakra is at the top of the forehead.*

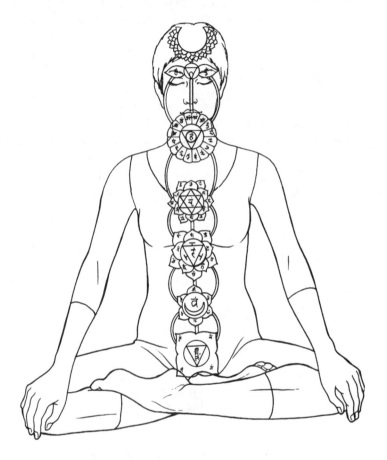

# *Kundalini Energy: Awakening Your Subtle Body*

*Kundalini* is the universe's creative energy. Although every person has kundalini, this energy lies in a state of rest, coiled snakelike at the base of your spine, until conscious efforts arouse and awaken it. When awakened, kundalini is like a supercharged lightning bolt of chi, coursing through your chakras to unite personal and cosmic energies within you. And once awakened, kundalini brings enlightenment, transcendence, and deep joy.

# Base Support: Energizing the Root Chakra

The first or root chakra houses kundalini (which you'll notice corresponds to the organs of fertility, your ovaries). Awakening and stimulating your kundalini energy awakens all of your chakras. Meditation, yoga, massage, and forms of bodywork such as Reiki can awaken kundalini. Significant events in your life—childbirth, a crisis, or extraordinary sex—can also trigger the release of kundalini. Most people recognize this release, even if they call it something different. By using techniques that connect your body and mind (yoga or meditation), you can learn to release kundalini energy as you need it to recharge and refresh your chakras and restore harmony to your body.

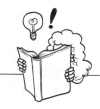

**Wise Up**

**Kundalini** is the most powerful of the energies contained in the chakras and resides within the first chakra. The word *kundalini* means "coiled like a snake" in Sanskrit.

### Meditation Exercise: Cleansing and Opening Your Chakras

The stress and pressure of everyday living can tarnish and block your chakras. Meditation is one method to cleanse your chakras, opening them to free the flow of chi. This meditation exercise is both easy and effective.

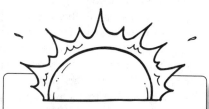

**Embracing Change**

For more about meditation and yoga, see *The Complete Idiot's Guide to Meditation* (Alpha Books, 1998) and *The Complete Idiot's Guide to Yoga* (Alpha Books, 1998), both by Joan Budilovsky and Eve Adamson.

1. Sit in a comfortable, open position, with no parts of your body crossing or blocking other parts.

2. Take several slow, deep breaths. Bring cleansing air deep into your lungs. Feel stress and tension leave your body each time that you exhale.

3. Starting with your root chakra, create a vision of what each chakra looks like. Focus on this image. Can you see the chakra's color? Does it vibrate and spin? Is it vivid and strong? If not (and if you're new to this meditation, it probably won't be—don't panic, because you're going to fix that), concentrate on cleaning it up until it shines bright and clear.

4. Follow the same process for each of your chakras, from root to crown. Picture each chakra filling with chi as you finish your cleansing and prepare to move to the next chakra.

5. When all seven chakras are clear and open, envision a strong current of chi coursing through them. Feel this energy pulse and spin as it activates the physical and psychic centers that each chakra regulates.

6. To draw your meditation to an end, again take several deep, slow breaths. Feel your chi settle into a harmonized, steady rhythm.

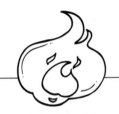

**Hot Flash!**

If you're new to yoga, consider enrolling in a class so that you can learn the postures correctly. Although yoga appears to be a mild form of exercise, many postures require much practice. If any yoga posture that you're attempting causes pain, stop immediately.

# Yoga to Strengthen, Lengthen, and Revitalize

Yoga combines physical postures with meditation. This ancient form of exercise helps tone and stretch your muscles, improves your balance, and clarifies your thought processes. Yoga also smoothes the flow of chi by stimulating your chakras. Various yoga postures activate different chakras. Nearly everyone can do some form of yoga.

You can practice yoga alone or with others in a yoga class. Taking a class is a great way to learn how to do yoga postures safely, to reduce your risk of injury. Yoga works to balance the energy of your endocrine system (which produces the hormones that are now driving you crazy). By stretching and toning your muscles, yoga provides the same benefit as other forms of physical exercise for helping to stabilize hormonal fluctuations (see Chapter 25, "Exercise: Menopause Magic").

**Yoga Posture for Menopause Relief: Downward-Facing Dog**

The yoga posture known as Downward-Facing Dog helps you to focus and direct energy inward. To do this posture, follow these steps:

1. Start on your hands and knees.

2. Raise your tailbone up as though you were starting to stand, using your toes to push yourself into position.

3. At the same time that your backside is rising, lower your head between your arms to make your back a straight line from tailbone to the top of your head.

4. Lower your heels until they're touching the floor. Straighten your knees as much as you can (if it hurts, stop).

5. Your weight should be balanced between your heels and your hands.

6. Hold this posture for as long as it is comfortable, and then slowly reverse your movements to return to your hands and knees.

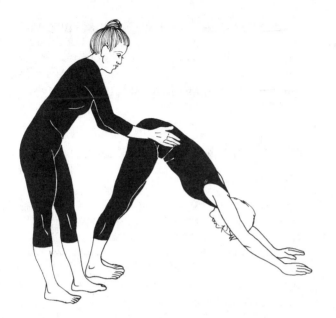

*Yoga's Downward-Facing Dog pose.*

# Meditate and Relax ... Yes, You!

*Meditation* can be a path to inner enlightenment as well as to outer relaxation. Many forms of meditation exist, from the traditional Buddhist *mantra* style to prayer and simple conscious awareness. Meditation can be a means for connecting your individual consciousness with the collective cosmos, or a form of communication with your deity of choice. It can be a physical action—walking a labyrinth (described a little later in this chapter), using prayer or rosary beads, or taking up yoga postures. Meditation can be as formal or as casual as you like, as long as the process that you choose to follow is purposeful and intentional. (In other words, you can't watch TV and call it meditation.)

Meditation is relaxing because it frees you from the thoughts that trouble you. It allows you to focus instead on an image or a sound, or even a particular thought, clearing all others from your mind. Once cleared, your mind can become calm and peaceful. When practiced regularly, meditation is a great way to relieve stress and tension that affects both your mind and your body.

### Wise Up

**Meditation** is a method for relaxing your body and your mind by consciously focusing on certain thoughts, objects, or sounds with the intent of excluding all others. A **mantra** is a sound or a combination of sounds that you make when you meditate, with the purpose of stimulating certain chakras or energies.

Your meditation sessions don't have to be long—just 10 or 15 minutes might be enough. And you don't need a special place or any special equipment, although many people like to use a space that they've set aside just for this purpose. If you do this, you can use candles, incense, and music to enhance your meditation sessions. But, if you're a seasoned meditator, you can also meditate on the bus on the way to work, in the park at lunchtime, or in your office on a break.

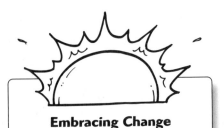

**Embracing Change**

Don't worry about whether you're meditating the "right" way. There are no right or wrong ways to meditate. Do what comes naturally.

# Finding Your Place in the Universe

Just as your menopause journey is a transition, it is also a quest. You are moving from one state of existence to another. It's natural to ask questions that you may not have pondered since adolescence. Who am I? Why am I here? What have I accomplished on this excursion that is my life, and what is left for me yet to accomplish? You're likely to come closer to answers that satisfy you than you did some 30-odd years ago. You have more wisdom and experience than that distant teenage self. You also might have a stronger sense of urgency, a more intense need to know—and a more confident belief that there is a something beyond your individual existence.

## *Menopause Mandalas*

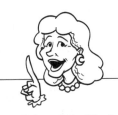

**Wise Woman's Wisdom**

"It is important to know that life is vital, and one's own living a torn fragment of the larger cloth."

—Marjorie Kinnan Rawlings

Many people use mandalas when they meditate. These objects, usually two-dimensional drawings, feature a pattern and elements that have meaning for you. Someone else's mandala may be just another pretty picture, while yours instantly triggers a process of insightful self-exploration. Mandalas are often connected to Buddhist monks, who painstakingly create elaborate designs of colored sand and then brush them away, symbolizing the transitory nature of existence. But mandalas have penetrated Western thinking, too. The psychoanalyst Carl Jung, most famous for his work in dream interpretation, viewed a mandala as a vessel into which an individual projected his or her psyche as a blend of psychology and spirituality.

It's easy to make your own mandala. You may find that you like to use different mandalas for various kinds of meditation or to stimulate specific chakras when you meditate. If you're new to mandalas, try a pattern of basic geometric designs, such as three overlapping circles or a square with a triangle inside of it. More complex mandalas feature various geometric shapes as well as representations of concepts or ideas that are important to you.

## Walking the Labyrinth: Purposeful Patterns

A *labyrinth* is a pattern with a purpose. It has only one path, although it may wind through many convolutions on its way to the center. The path leading into the labyrinth is a path of release. As you follow it, you begin to leave your worries and concerns behind. When you reach the labyrinth's center, you experience illumination or enlightenment. The path leading out of the labyrinth (the same path you followed in) helps you integrate your experiences so that you can grow from them after you leave the labyrinth. For most people, walking a labyrinth is a powerful emotional and spiritual experience. Although you may not have access to a labyrinth you can walk through, you can easily draw a miniature labyrinth that you can trace with your finger.

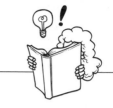

**Wise Up**

A **labyrinth** is a single, or unicursal, path that follows a number of circuits before ending up in the center. To leave, you follow the path back again. In contrast, a maze presents multiple (multicursal) paths and numerous choices. The way in and the way out are often different.

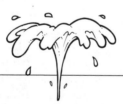

**Wellspring**

In the thirteenth century, leaders of the Chartres Cathedral in Paris inlaid an intricate pattern of blue and white stone tiles in the floor of the nave, or center of worship. People came to the cathedral to walk the labyrinth that the pattern created, just as they made pilgrimages to Lourdes and other places of faith. The winding stone trail leading to the labyrinth's center symbolized the wanderings along life's path, and the steady spiritual guidance keeping life on track. Today, millions of people in all cultures use variations of the Chartres labyrinth for spiritual and emotional healing.

*The famous labyrinth at Chartres Cathedral. Use a pencil to trace the sacred pattern.*

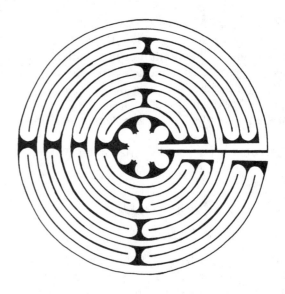

Walking a labyrinth is a powerful healing experience. Many hospitals have labyrinths on their grounds for patients, families, and staff to use. A labyrinth is particularly helpful for leading you to clarity in times of transition. Some people meditate or pray as they follow the labyrinth's twists and turns. Others find solace and peace in the steady and repetitive pattern of following the labyrinth's winding paths.

As you trace or walk a labyrinth, resist the urge to rush ahead or cross over the boundaries to get to the finish. It's the journey that matters. Just let the path lead you, as a symbolic representation of how the path of your life leads you. When you reach the center, stay for a while. Contemplate, meditate, pray, and think. Allow yourself to join with the bigger scheme. Then turn around and follow the path back out. Just as your finger traces this pattern on paper (or your feet walk its path), your life follows its own path and pattern. While your personal labyrinth is unique to you, it is also itself part of a larger labyrinth, another of the cycles of existence.

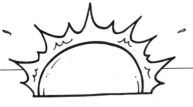

### Embracing Change

Because your mandala is a personal symbol, you can make it as simple or as complex as you choose. When you use your mandala as a meditation guide, it should help you feel a sense of inner calm and order, even if your thoughts wander as you're looking at it. If you feel anxious, annoyed, or frustrated, try a different mandala.

# Tapping Ovarian Wisdom

Nothing in nature exists without purpose. The flower that blossoms becomes the seed of new life, and the new life draws energy from the seed that has now become its sustenance. Even when old life ends, it returns to the soil to continue nurturing and nourishing. It is the labyrinth of life, the circle of chi, and the cycle of existence. As the gardens that produce the seeds of human life, your ovaries symbolize both the physiological and the spiritual dimensions of existence.

## The Energy of Life: Ovarian Chi

Researchers want to find the physiological functions that appear to stimulate the burst of creative expression that many women feel at menopause. When they can identify these functions, they believe that they'll be able to explain the mysteries of menopause's emotional and spiritual shifts. And good evidence exists to support the role that hormones play in altering your brain's neurotransmitters. But is this the entire answer? Intuitively, we have to say no. Looking again at the bigger scheme, there's an enormous shift of energy that takes place at menopause as well.

All of your adult life, your ovaries nurture the potential of new life. Their energy focuses outward, guiding the sequence of physical and emotional events to prepare you for your role in this possibility. Month after month, year after year, the cycle repeats, following an internal labyrinth to its center and back out again. Then at menopause, the cycle slows. As hormone levels drop, your ovaries bring to an end your ability to generate new life.

From a *metaphysical* perspective, it's not just hormone levels that change. At menopause, your ovarian energy reverses. Instead of preparing for prospective life, your ovaries turn their focus to nourishing the life that already exists: yours. Yes, hormone production drops way off. But it doesn't stop entirely, and what remains continues to serve vital functions for your body. (Even if scientists can't entirely pin this down, they know it to be true.) Yes, you experience the loss of fertility, but you remain a dynamic and creative life force. And now, that creativity and energy can feed your existence.

> **Wise Up**
>
> **Metaphysical** means beyond or around the physical. It's a term that typically encompasses experiences that involve the body, mind, and spirit as a collective whole.

## Ovarian Energy and the New, Creative You

Many women experience a burst of creative energy when ovarian function shifts its focus away from fertility. It's no coincidence that midlife is often a time of artistic expression. You might decide to take up watercolor painting, write a novel, compose a musical score, act in local theater, or choreograph a dance. Your opportunities for enjoying your newfound creative energy are endless.

# Finding Center

As with any time of transition, you're likely to feel unsettled and off-center during menopause. You're not going crazy, we promise. Although you can't force the path or pattern of your menopause journey, you can guide your body, mind, and spirit toward unity and calm. Use meditation, yoga, bodywork, massage, and other tools to help recenter yourself. Then you can willingly follow the path of your journey and be comfortable in knowing that it will take you where you need to go.

---

### The Least You Need to Know

➤ Your menopause journey is but one of many paths through life. Like a labyrinth, it can be complex and circuitous, but it will always lead you to the center.

➤ Awakening the energy of your chakras can help you make more sense out of the experiences that you're having.

➤ Kundalini is like supercharged chi that can enrich and invigorate your body, mind, and spirit.

➤ Use the labyrinth as a tool for self-discovery as well as for problem-solving.

➤ Meditation is a great stress-reliever. You can meditate just about anywhere.

---

# Part 7

# Vibrant, Feminine, Wise, and Wonderful

*It's a new you—wholesome, invigorated, and ready to enjoy life to the fullest. Now the only challenge that remains is how to keep your body and mind primed for good health. Yes, there are some potential bumps in the road. But there are also actions that you can take to prevent them from blocking your path. Take good care of your body, and it will take good care of you.*

*These last chapters discuss the many ways that you can improve your well-being and monitor your health.*

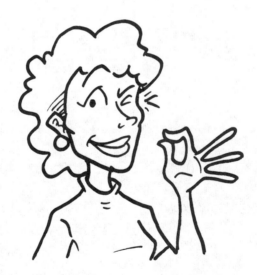

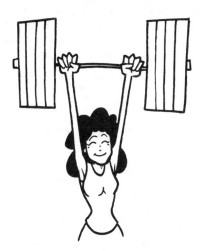

# Chapter 25

# Exercise: Menopause Magic

## In This Chapter

➤ The relationship between long life and exercise

➤ What's your fitness level? A self-quiz

➤ Adding physical activity to your everyday life

➤ Why exercise is especially important during your menopause transition

➤ Why the exercise you get now is more important than the exercise you got (or didn't get) when you were younger

Can help for your menopause discomforts be as close as a pair of running shoes? Many health experts believe so. Exercise appears to have positive effects on a wide range of menopause problems, from hot flashes to sleep disturbances. We're not talking about running marathons, either. Just 30 minutes of exercise a day, four or five days a week, can work like a magic elixir to ease the effects of your erratic hormones.

Even if you're already active, you can find comfort in structured exercise. Much of the activity that engages us throughout the busy day is purposeful yet frantic, and doesn't extend for long enough to benefit our bodies. Planned, regular exercise—even just walking—can relieve stress, control weight, and strengthen muscles and bones.

## Nature Knows

The human body is made for movement. Your musculoskeletal system—bones, muscles, and connective tissues—is a marvel of levers, pivots, and hinges. Muscles, tendons, and ligaments stretch and relax in opposition to one another, permitting you to twist, turn, jump, reach, and transport yourself from one location to another. No other design of nature features such complexity or autonomy. This body of yours can carry you through decades of active living, even if you never give its capabilities a second thought. Just imagine what your body could do if you actually *did* think about its capabilities!

## How to Live to Be a Healthy 100: Exercise

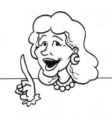

**Wise Woman's Wisdom**

"It's not how old you are, but how you are old."

—Marie Dressler

A friend just celebrated her 96th birthday. When asked what she's done to stay healthy and vital for so many years, she says simply, "When I feel tired, I go for a walk." People who live long are people whose lives are active and full. Many were mothers and wives for most of their adult lives, raising families and keeping house in a time when if you didn't do it yourself, it didn't get done. Although they could relax and let today's modern conveniences take over some of the more demanding tasks, they choose not to. They still walk to the mailbox, work in the garden, climb the stairs, and wash floors. That's not a workout by contemporary standards, perhaps, but their bodies need the constant level of exercise to stay in prime operating condition.

## Exercise and the Human Life Span

A baby born today can reasonably hope to live to be 80 or 90 years old. Whether she realizes this potential will depend a lot on how she chooses to live her life. All other factors not withstanding, a life of activity and exercise will continue to carry future generations toward long and healthy lives. But what about you? Research shows that the more active you are, the more likely it is that you can hold off many of the health problems that can threaten your longevity and the quality of your life, including diabetes, many forms of cancer, and, of course, our familiar enemies by now: heart disease and osteoporosis. Exercise is truly the fountain of youth.

## Whatever You Do, Keep Moving

Once you get going, it doesn't take a lot to keep your body moving. You have dozens of opportunities each day to stretch and flex your muscles. Park your car at the back of the lot so that you can walk to the store or the office. Take the stairs instead of the elevator. Pace whatever distance your telephone cord will allow when you're trapped on the phone. Fidget when you're watching television or sitting in front of the computer. Every move you make adds up.

# Fitness Level? What Fitness Level?

What's your fitness level? Everyone has one (even if you haven't seen yours for some time now). In technical terms, your fitness level is the ability of your body to manage physical activities requiring endurance and strength. A person who gets regular physical exercise usually has a high fitness level, while someone who seldom gets off her seat generally has a low fitness level. But take heart—your fitness level is one of the few things in life that's actually easy to raise.

## *Exercise and You: A Self-Quiz*

What kind of exercise do you do right now? How much time do you spend doing it? Is it enough to do your body any good? Here are a few quick questions to help you get a handle on your fitness level.

1. The farthest distance that you might walk in a day is ...

    **a.** From the car to the door.

    **b.** A few blocks, if you count walking back and forth all day.

    **c.** A mile or more.

2. When you bend forward from the waist, how far can you reach without turning red in the face?

    **a.** Knees.

    **b.** Ankles or toes.

    **c.** Beyond ... to the floor.

3. If a gust of wind blows a dollar bill out of your hand, you ...

    **a.** Wave goodbye.

    **b.** Try to stomp on it with your foot.

    **c.** Give chase.

4. If you have to stop at the grocery store on your way home to pick up a few things for dinner, where do you park?

    **a.** Along the curb in the fire zone—you won't be in the store that long.

    **b.** In the first regular parking space that you find.

    **c.** At the back of the parking lot so that you can stretch your legs.

5. Your kids or grandkids want to go for a bicycle ride. You ...

    **a.** Help them fasten their helmets and kiss them goodbye.

    **b.** Walk up and down the sidewalk as they ride up and down the street.

    **c.** Grab your helmet and bike and race them to the corner.

6. Your car is so dirty that you can't tell what color it is. You ...
   a. Take it to the automatic carwash.
   b. Get the soap and rags ready, and then pay your kids, grandkids, or the neighbor kids to wash while you rinse.
   c. Put on your work clothes, and give it a thorough wash and wax.

7. You find yourself with a half-hour of unexpected free time in the middle of the afternoon. You ...
   a. Take a nap.
   b. Go shopping.
   c. Lace up your tennies and do a few laps around the block.

Give yourself five points for each c, three points for each b, and one point for each a. If your total is 30 or more, treat yourself to a walk after dinner tonight—you're probably in pretty good shape. If your total is between 21 and 29, you could use some more workout time, but you can probably take the stairs when the elevator's slow or out of order. If your total is 20 or less, you need to get moving!

## Getting Started When You've Never Exercised

One challenge for many women is that even though the health experts may consider your lifestyle to be a sedentary one, you're far from inactive. Your life is busy from the instant you wake up until the moment you fall back into bed again, 16 or 18 hours later. Where are you supposed to find the time to add exercise to your day? Well, start by taking a look at all the many tasks and responsibilities that occupy your time. How many actually require your participation? Sometimes giving up time is like giving up control. But really, you're gaining the power to influence and change your own life.

Start small. Take 10 minutes in the morning to walk up and down the stairs. If you can't bring yourself to do something that has no outcome, carry laundry or papers or books with you. There's always something downstairs that needs to go upstairs, and vice versa. Take another 10 minutes at lunch to walk out the door and to the corner. Take a deep breath. Isn't it great to be out in the fresh air? Turn around and come back, if you must, or continue around the block. Call it a stress break.

Once these simple activities become comfortable, move on to bigger things. Dust off your bicycle and go for a ride after dinner. Call a friend and go walking around the track at a nearby high school or through a local park. Enroll in a Wednesday evening aerobic dance class or swim program. A few hours one evening a week won't force any sacrifices, will it? Once you get moving, you'll be surprised at how you look forward to these daily activities—and how amazing it is to recognize that the health experts call them exercise!

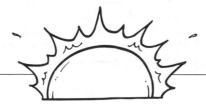

### Embracing Change

Is your life just too busy for exercise? According to the American Heart Association, you have 336 opportunities each week to get in 30 minutes' worth of exercise. That's how many 30-minute blocks of time there are in a week. Surely you can use three or four of them for your good health!

You can join a health club or start a weight-training program, if you want (although you don't have to do this to get a good workout). Most communities have a number of organizations that sponsor physical activities for mature adults, from ballroom dancing to rock climbing. Choose activities that appeal to you. Try things you've always wanted to do but haven't ever had the money, the time, or the guts.

## Ask Your Doctor First

How long has it been since physical activity quickened your heart rate and deepened your breathing? If more than six months, start your regular exercise plan with a checkup from your doctor. This will give you a clear idea of your starting point and will help you accommodate any unique physical needs that you might have.

## Tracking Your Progress

It's natural to look for obvious signs that your commitment to exercise is paying off. Most of us want to look in the mirror or at the scale for this evidence, viewing exercise as a tool for weight loss as much as anything else. Although losing a few pounds is a pleasant inevitability for many women who begin exercising after a long hiatus of physical inactivity, it's not the measure that matters. And, in fact, it's possible to improve your overall health and fitness and actually *gain* a few pounds. This is because muscle weighs more than fat.

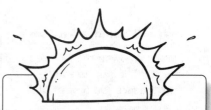

### Embracing Change

Ask a friend or your partner to join you in your physical activities. Studies show that people are far more likely to continue an active lifestyle if they have someone to share in their efforts.

Two measures that do count are body mass index (BMI) and waist-to-hip ratio. For a refresher on BMI, page back to Chapter 20, "Nutrition: Eating Your Way Through a Healthy Menopause." While BMI addresses health risks in general, waist-to-hip ratio reflects your risk for heart disease. To measure your waist-to-hip ratio, you need a flexible tape measure (the kind you use for sewing, not the kind you use for measuring lumber).

1. Stand with your feet together. Relax so that you're not sucking your belly in.

2. Wrap the tape measure securely, but not tightly, around the center of your body (between your navel and your hips), and write down the measurement in inches.

3. Next, wrap the tape measure securely, but not tightly, around the widest point of your hips. Record this measurement, in inches.

4. Divide your waist measurement by your hip measurement. This gives the ratio between your waist and your hips. For example, if your waist is 28 inches and your hips measure 38 inches, your waist-to-hip ratio is 0.736, or 74 percent.

For women over age 50, waist size should be no more than 80 percent of your hip measurement, which is a ratio of 0.8 or less. A ratio greater than this suggests an accumulation of body fat around your middle that could be a warning sign that you are at risk for heart disease.

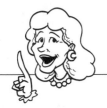

**Wise Woman's Wisdom**

"Nature gives you the face you have at 20; it is up to you to merit the face you have at 50."

—Coco Chanel

Human nature being what it is, we all want to see evidence that our efforts produce results. But focusing on weight loss as a measure of fitness is like looking at the bark of a tree to gauge its height. You have to step back and look at the bigger picture. And you'll probably never actually see the most significant improvements, which are on the inside. You should notice their reflections, however, in how you feel—energetic, alert, calm, and at peace with your world. You'll also be able to climb stairs, run for the bus, or walk through the airport instead of taking the moving sidewalks, all without appearing like you've just completed a marathon.

# Movin' and Menopause

Imagine for a moment that you're riding a bicycle. It's an older bicycle, maybe one that doesn't shift so smoothly any more, but still a strong and functional bicycle. Now think of the air in your bicycle's tires. If the air pressure is too low, the tires are mushy and soft. They'll roll, but only with considerable effort. The sides balloon out, drooping to drag along the road. Steering and turning are possible but sluggish. Pump up the air pressure, and a marvelous transformation takes place. The tires become firm and alert. With far less rubber in contact with the road, they roll smoothly and confidently. The bicycle responds to your every action, holding its course and steering almost as if it can read your mind.

Exercising is like putting air in your tires. It pumps up your cells so that they're primed for peak performance. As your body gets older, its "tires" don't hold air as well as when it was younger. You need to pump it up regularly to keep it running smoothly and efficiently. But if you do this, it will carry you where you want to go for a long, long time.

## Special Benefits of Exercise During Perimenopause

Perimenopause is that awkward stage of "not quite." Your menstrual cycles are not quite regular, but they haven't quite come to an end. You may have both PMS and hot flashes. Your hormones don't know which way they're going—up this month, down next month. What's a woman to do? Although exercise might not be the first thought that comes to mind, it's one of the easiest and most effective ways to tame and level your body's imbalances. (No, peeling the wrapper from a chocolate bar doesn't count as exercise.) Because exercise increases your metabolism, it helps your cells to function more efficiently. They'll still respond to fluctuating hormones, but they can do so more quickly.

Exercise during perimenopause also slows the loss of calcium from your bones, which is an important factor in preventing osteoporosis. Beginning at about age 35, your body starts to lose its ability to draw calcium from the foods that you eat (including supplements). You need to take in more, even as your body uses less. Estrogen plays a role in calcium loss, too. Weight-bearing activities such as walking, jogging, or sports such as tennis or racquetball help keep your bones stronger and healthier.

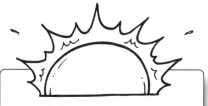

**Embracing Change**

How do you know if you're exercising at the right level for fitness? If you can sing while you exercise, you need to pick up the pace. If you can barely wheeze out your name, you're working too hard. But if you can exercise and carry on a conversation, your efforts are probably on target.

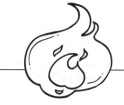

**Hot Flash!**

If you still smoke, this is an ideal time to kick the habit. Cigarette smoking is the leading cause of heart disease, making it a companion that you could live without when your risk for heart disease increases following menopause.

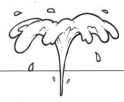

**Wellspring**

The American Heart Association (AHA) sponsors an online physical activity program for women called "Choose to Move." This free program is designed to get you moving for at least 30 minutes a day most days of the week. This is the level that the AHA research shows is effective in reducing your risk for heart disease and stroke. You start gradually, with activities that your personal fitness level can sustain. Each week for 12 weeks you'll receive information, suggestions, and recommended activities designed to move you toward your fitness goals. More than 24,000 women participated in "Choose to Move" in 1999. For more information, visit the program's Web site at www.justmove.org.

## Special Benefits of Exercise During Menopause

Once you're clearly on your menopause journey—no doubts about those hot flashes, and PMS now means "power for myself"—the benefits of exercise continue to multiply. Exercise gives your cells the power to use what little estrogen, progesterone, and testosterone comes their way to maximum advantage. This can curb hot flashes and stabilize mood swings. Regular exercise can improve your sex drive and help you sleep better at night (which are not mutually exclusive). And exercise just makes you feel better, in part because it releases those feel-good substances that your body saves for special occasions, endorphins.

## Special Benefits of Exercise After Menopause

During the first two or three years following menopause—that retrospective date, now at least a year behind you, when you had your last period—your risk for heart disease increases at a faster rate than at any other time in your life. Regular exercise is your key to maintaining heart health during this time of particular challenge. It reduces blood cholesterol levels, lowers blood pressure, and strengthens your heart muscle. As an element of your everyday life, exercise can help keep your risk for heart disease as low as possible for decades following menopause. Regular exercise also lowers your risk for health conditions such as diabetes and improves your balance and flexibility, reducing your risk of injury due to falls.

# Fly Like a Butterfly, Sting Like a Bee

A fit body is a masterpiece of deception. It makes every movement look effortless and smooth—which it might be, for a finely tuned body. But keeping that body in prime condition takes more than wishful thinking. You don't have to become a fixture at the health club, but you do need to incorporate regular exercise into your daily life. Boxing great Muhammad Ali has a wonderful quote about the value of experience through age: "The man [or woman!] who views the world at 50 the same as he did at 20 has wasted 30 years of his [her!] life."

## Use It or Lose It

The best way to keep your body in good working order is to keep it working. Regular activity tones and strengthens muscles and bones, improves circulation, and even gives your skin that healthy glow. Exercise restores flexibility and movement, making it a great way to manage chronic problems such as back pain or arthritis. If you don't use it, you will lose it—and you could reach a point at which you can't get it back anymore. If you've been an on-again, off-again exerciser, this isn't news to you. Even though it may take several weeks to get your body in shape, it takes only a few days of inactivity for it to begin slipping out of shape again.

## The Late Bloom Lasts Longest

Recent research shows that you gain significant health benefits from regular exercise no matter how old you are when you start. Doctors have long believed that people who engaged in regular, moderate to intensive exercise during their 20s and 30s built up a savings account of benefits that carried through later decades. We now know that although this is still true, the interest rate isn't as high as we thought. It's the exercise that you're doing right now that seems to have the greatest protective benefit for your health.

Exercise at any time of your life has both immediate and future benefits, of course, and we're certainly not discouraging or disparaging exercise while you're younger. But you gain the most from steady, consistent activity over time—all the time. And health benefits are greater if you start exercising at age 40 or 50 and continue for the rest of your life than if you exercised strenuously through your 20s and 30s and then slack off at midlife.

## The Least You Need to Know

➤ Your body needs regular physical activity to function at (and look) its best.

➤ Fitness is not about weight loss, although losing weight may be a pleasant result of your fitness efforts. Fitness is about creating a healthy environment to support your body and your life.

➤ Although more is better to a point, just 30 minutes a day for four or five days every week is enough exercise to tone and strengthen your body.

➤ Exercise can provide both short-term relief from menopause discomforts and long-term protection from health problems related to estrogen loss, such as heart disease and osteoporosis.

➤ Many everyday activities can exercise your body, including walking, climbing stairs, gardening, and doing housework.

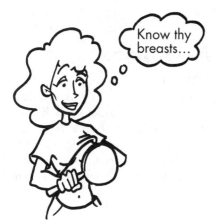

# Chapter 26

# Staying Healthy After Menopause: Outer Changes

---

**In This Chapter**

➤ What routine gynecological care is important after menopause

➤ Why pelvic exams are so important after menopause

➤ How you can lower your risk for cervical cancer

➤ How to examine your breasts

➤ What to do if you find a lump in your breast

---

Although the dramatic events that mark your menopause transition come to a close once menopause is complete, your body continues to change as it adjusts to its new hormonal environment. These changes take place at a much slower pace than the whirlwind of changes that you've just experienced, but they will continue for the rest of your life as your body's tissues fine-tune their functions.

You'll see outward evidence of some of these changes: Collagen and connective tissues lose elasticity, for example, producing those characteristic laugh lines around your mouth and your eyes. (Okay, you can call them crow's feet if you choose, but we prefer a more upbeat perspective.) Breast, uterine, and vaginal tissues change as well. Although most of these changes are harmless, some can have serious health consequences, such as cancer.

This chapter discusses these more obvious outward signs of life after menopause. Evidence of other changes is more subtle and may not show itself until fully dressed in the garb of health problems such as heart disease and osteoporosis. We discuss these consequences of menopause in Chapter 27, "Staying Healthy After Menopause: Inner Changes."

# The Female Body-Mind *After* Menopause

For the vast majority of women, the discomforts of the menopause journey come to a close at the trail's end. For a small percentage of women, however, the signs do continue after menopause concludes, especially hot flashes, although doctors aren't sure why. If you are among these exceptional women, discuss your situation with your doctor to be sure that there aren't underlying physical reasons. The same treatments and therapies that provided relief during your menopause journey can still help now. And you'll probably want to revisit your HRT decision, especially to consider starting HRT if you've not yet done so.

## What's Happening Inside Your Body

For most women, life settles down after menopause. Your hormones stabilize at the levels that they will maintain for the rest of your life, and your tissues and organ systems have already begun to adapt. Your new body is beginning to feel more like an old friend, and it no longer surprises you with hot flashes and other discomforts. Without the supply of estrogen that they've become accustomed to, however, many tissues continue to change.

## Calm After the Emotional Storm

Your mind is settling into its new environment, too. All those memory lapses and chaotic thoughts that caused you to wonder if you were about to lose your mind have evolved into a heightened state of awareness. You are more alert, insightful, intuitive, and creative. Your mood is generally stable (and often positive). You have become the wise woman.

# Routine GYN Care After Menopause

Maintaining your gynecological health after menopause should be a partnership between you and your healthcare provider. Some exams you should do yourself, and others your doctor should do. The more familiar you are with your body and how it looks and feels under ordinary circumstances, the better able you are to detect changes before they become health problems. In fact, at no time in your life has such regular monitoring been more important than it is now. As you grow older, your risk for many health problems naturally increases. Knowing when a change takes place gives you a tremendous advantage in heading off a potentially life-threatening challenge.

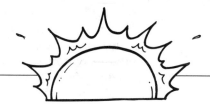

**Embracing Change**

To help you remember when your routine GYN care is due, get a calendar that you can use as your women's health calendar. Mark the day of each month that you do BSE (breast self-exam). Mark the dates you should have your pelvic exam and Pap test, mammogram, and any other care your gynecologist recommends. Hang the calendar in your bathroom or bedroom, where you'll see it every day.

# Pelvic Exams and Pap Tests

If you thought menopause meant an end to your time in the stirrups, we're sorry to break it to you: Your gynecologist's office is going to become a familiar place. Pelvic exams and *Pap tests* are more important now than they've ever been. These health screenings are your first line of defense against the potential health problems that become more common as you grow older.

**Wise Up**

A **Pap test,** named after the physician who invented it, Dr. George Papanicolaou, detects cancerous cells scraped from the surface of the cervix.

A typical pelvic exam includes manual palpation (examination by touch) of your external genitalia, vagina, cervix, ovaries, and rectum. Your gynecologist will scrape some cells from your cervix for a Pap test (a painless procedure that takes just a few seconds) and also will examine your breasts. It's helpful to schedule your regular mammogram, if you have one, to take place a few weeks before your GYN visit so that your doctor can discuss the results with you. Women age 50 and older should have a pelvic exam and a Pap test each year. If you've had cervical cancer, human papilloma virus infections (HPV, or genital warts), or other gynecological problems, your gynecologist may recommend more frequent exams.

## Uterus Redux

Ah, here it is again, that pesky uterus of yours. Just when diminishing periods lead you to believe that this womb is closed for business, here we are to remind you that even though you don't see evidence of its presence any longer, your uterus still needs

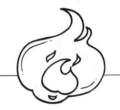

**Hot Flash!**

You should still have regular pelvic exams and Pap tests even if you've had a hysterectomy. Although you no longer have to worry about endometrial (uterine) cancer, other potential health risks still exist.

your regular attention. If you're not taking HRT, your uterus will continue to shrink until it becomes a shadow of its former self. It has no further functions, and usually it presents no problems. However, there is a chance—fairly slim—that it could become a site for cancer to develop.

Estrogen replacement can act like a fertilizer for endometrial cancer, providing a rich environment for cancer cells to take root and grow. If you have your uterus and are taking HRT, you're most likely taking progesterone to counter this risk. Although a few women may continue to experience periodic bleeding with HRT, most women no longer bleed after menopause. If you again have vaginal bleeding, have your gynecologist check it out. Regular GYN exams are also a good way to monitor for changes.

## Cervical Cancer

Cervical cancer once killed 20,000 women a year. Then routine Pap tests made it possible to diagnose this deadly disease in its earliest stages, and now cervical cancer claims the lives of fewer than 5,000 women a year. Doctors believe that cervical cancer could soon be a disease of history, now that we know that a common virus—human papilloma virus, or HPV—causes 95 percent of all cases.

There are dozens of strains of HPV, several of which cause genital warts. Scientists now know that some of these strains of HPV cause up to 95 percent of all cases of cervical cancer. As a result, women who have had HPV infections have an increased risk for cervical cancer and should have annual Pap tests no matter what their ages. Currently there is no cure for HPV, although using condoms during sexual intercourse can prevent infection.

## Ovarian Cysts and Cancer Risks

Ovarian cysts are common—so common, in fact, that it's unlikely that there's a woman who hasn't had one (or won't get one) during her lifetime. Most ovarian cysts are harmless and are so quiet that you don't even know they're there. Spawned by your hormone cycle, they bubble from an ovarian follicle. Some reach 6 or 7 centimeters (about 2 inches) in diameter before they either rupture or recede. Ovarian cysts are not as likely to occur after menopause because your follicles are no longer producing eggs, although you can still get them. You might find one of these fluid-filled growths coincidentally, if you happen to have a pelvic exam or a pelvic ultrasound when one is present. Less commonly, you might discover that an ovarian cyst is to blame for pelvic discomfort.

There is no correlation between ovarian cysts and ovarian cancer. Most ovarian cancer develops in the thin tissue that covers the ovaries, called the epithelium. Some cancerous tumors also develop in the tissue that produces estrogen and progesterone, causing health experts to speculate that there is a relationship between menopause and ovarian cancer. Ovarian cancer is uncommon at any age, although it does increase after age 50. Unfortunately, there are few early signs of ovarian cancer, which is a key reason why ovarian cancer claims the lives of more than half the women who get it. Regular pelvic exams are crucial for early detection, which can catch the cancer before it spreads from the ovaries to other parts of the body.

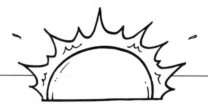

**Embracing Change**

Many women worry that pain in their breasts or lower pelvic area is a sign of cancer. Most often this is not the case. Most cancers are painless and unobtrusive until they become advanced, which is why preventive screenings are so important. By all means, have your doctor check out any pain that has a sudden and severe onset or that continues for longer than two weeks. But most pain, without other symptoms, is not cancer.

# Nurturing Breast Health

Your breasts are public evidence of your womanhood. Whatever their size and shape, they present living proof of your ability to nurture and sustain life (regardless of whether you've ever used them for this purpose). Their first major metamorphosis took place 40 years ago or so, when they blossomed from the buds of childhood. If you bore children, they morphed again into vessels of nourishment. And now your breasts are changing once again. Much of the fibrous tissue that was once necessary to support the intricate network of milk ducts gradually shrinks away, replaced by fatty tissue that isn't quite so buoyant. Although most of the effect is appearance, these changes also make your breasts more susceptible to invasion by abnormal cells that can produce cysts, tumors, and other growths.

## *How to Do a Breast Self-Exam (BSE)*

A *breast self-exam (BSE)* is the single most important measure that you can take to protect yourself from breast cancer. Women detect about 80 percent of all breast cancers themselves, often in their early, treatable stages. Fortunately, however, the majority of lumps that BSE turns up are benign (not cancerous). Your doctor might want to do further testing, such as a *mammogram* or a *biopsy*, to be sure.

**293**

## Wise Up

A **breast self-exam** (**BSE**) is a technique for you to systematically explore your breasts to feel for unusual lumps. A **mammogram** is an x-ray of your breasts. To do a **biopsy,** your doctor removes a small sample of suspicious tissue and sends it to a laboratory for analysis.

You should do a BSE every month. Because you no longer have menstruation as a reminder, choose a date that's easy for you to remember, such as the first day of the month. There are three steps to BSE: visual inspection, palpation while standing, and palpation while lying down. Unsure of your technique? Ask your primary care physician or your GYN to go through a BSE with you. Your doctor can answer your questions, help you improve your technique, and show you exactly what to look for and where to look for it. In the meantime, here's an overview of how to examine your breasts.

**BSE Step One: Visual Inspection**

Start by standing in front of a mirror without your top and bra.

➤ Look at your breasts. Although each may have a slightly different appearance, they should be symmetrical and balanced. Look for any areas of unusual dimpling or rippling.

➤ Simultaneously raise your arms above your head. Your breasts should move in unison.

➤ Become familiar with the appearance of your breasts so that you'll know if you see any changes.

**BSE Step Two: Palpation While Standing**

This step is easiest to do in the shower because your wet hands will glide more smoothly over the surface of your breasts.

➤ To examine your left breast, raise your left arm over your head.

➤ Move the fingers of your right hand along your breast. Use the fleshy pads at the ends of your fingers, not just your fingertips. Cover the entire surface of your breast, from under your arm and near your collarbone to the nipple.

➤ Move in a circular, wedge, or up-and-down pattern, and follow the same pattern each time that you do BSE. Use firm but gentle pressure (with too much pressure, you'll feel your ribs, which you might mistake for lumps).

➤ Switch to do the other breast, and repeat the process.

### BSE Step Three: Palpation While Lying Down

Lying down spreads out your breast tissue, providing a different perspective. Lie on your back on your bed or other flat surface.

➤ To examine your left breast, put your left arm above your head.

➤ As you did when standing, move your fingers along the entire surface of your breast.

➤ Switch to do the other breast, and repeat the process.

**Embracing Change**

Do you have breast implants? If so, you should still do regular BSEs. Implants typically go under your breast tissue, so you can still feel the natural you. And you can still develop breast cancer. Regular BSEs have the same benefits for you as for women without implants.

# If You Find a Lump in Your Breast

Because early treatment is essential for the best outcome with breast cancer, have your doctor immediately evaluate any breast lump that you detect. If it's nothing, great. You and your doctor will both be relieved. And if it is cancer, you've given yourself the best chance for full recovery.

The vast majority of breast lumps—probably 90 percent or more—turn out to be something other than cancer. Many are fluid-filled cysts that either go away on their own or can be aspirated (your doctor uses a narrow needle to suck the fluid from the cyst so that it collapses and becomes reabsorbed). Other common forms of breast lumps include fibroadenomas, which feel rather rubbery and unattached, and changes due to fibrocystic breast syndrome, which is a common but harmless condition in which breast tissue becomes granular and lumpy.

Sometimes calcium deposits cause breast lumps. These lumps feel firm and attached. Calcium deposits are more common as you get older, although no one knows for sure why they occur. Because some forms of breast cancer draw calcium into them, most doctors will order a mammogram to evaluate the calcium pattern (the calcium within a cancerous tumor has a unique and distinctive pattern). If there is any doubt, your gynecologist will biopsy or remove the lump.

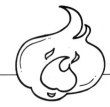

**Hot Flash!**

Have your doctor immediately evaluate any lumps or distortions that you find in your breasts. Early detection and treatment are essential if it is cancer. Don't wait; don't just *think* and *worry* about it; and, especially, don't *ignore* it. This is not a time to be Scarlett O'Hara and "think about it tomorrow." Go see your doctor right away!

Many women wonder just how they'd know if something they feel is a lump or just typical breast tissue. After all, breasts are somewhat lumpy by nature, and each woman's lumps are uniquely hers. With BSE, you're not necessarily looking for lumps so much as something different in the way that your breasts look or feel. This is the advantage of doing BSE every month—you develop an intimate familiarity with your breasts. You know what's normal for you. Some gynecologists have models made of materials that feel realistically like breast tissue to demonstrate variations in what's normal as well as what a suspicious lump might feel like.

## What Does a Mammogram Tell You?

A mammogram is an x-ray of your breast. Normal breast tissue is not very dense, meaning that it doesn't show up very well on an x-ray. Cancerous tumors, on the other hand, often contain calcium. This makes them more dense than normal breast tissue, so they do show up.

Mammograms can be preventive or diagnostic. Preventive, or screening, mammograms are those that you receive annually (or according to the intervals recommended for your age and health history). Your doctor isn't looking for anything specific, just anything that might appear unusual. A diagnostic mammogram is looking for something specific. Perhaps you or your doctor felt a lump in your breast. A mammogram can provide additional information about how far the lump extends into your breast tissue and whether the pattern of its growth suggests a malignancy (cancerous tumor). This is helpful for your doctor to know in case she decides to do a *biopsy*. A mammogram alone cannot determine whether a lump is cancer, however.

## Should You Have Screening Mammograms?

Health experts disagree about when and how often a woman should get screening mammograms. The American Cancer Society recommends annual screening mammograms for women age 40 and older. Other health experts recommend a baseline mammogram sometime between age 40 and 50, with annual screening mammograms after age 50. And some health experts believe that screening mammograms are of little value in discovering breast cancer because only one or two out of every 1,000 detect a cancerous tumor.

So what should you do? The answer depends on a number of factors, including whether you've completed menopause and if you're at increased risk for developing breast cancer. Before menopause, your breast tissue is fairly dense and fibrous. Although it's not as dense as bone, it still shows up on an x-ray. Unfortunately, this makes it difficult for the radiologist to determine whether there are abnormal growths in your breasts. After menopause, breast tissue changes from fibrous to fatty, making it easier to spot tumors.

In the end, the decision about whether to have annual screening mammograms is between you and your doctor. The primary risks are unnecessary biopsies and anxiety because of false-positive results. The benefit is that mammography can detect tumors that are still too small for you to feel or that are in locations where they'd be hard to feel.

## Breast Cancer Risks

All factors being equal, you have a 1 in 12 chance of developing breast cancer at some time in your life, if you live to age 85. Breast cancer is less common before age 40, and it becomes increasingly more common with each decade after age 40. The exception is for hereditary breast cancer, which accounts for about 5 percent of all cases of breast cancer. You may be at increased risk for breast cancer if you answer "yes" to two or more of these questions:

➤ Have two or more close relatives (mother, sisters, daughters) had breast cancer?

➤ Have family members been diagnosed with breast cancer before age 50?

➤ Have family members with breast cancer had the disease diagnosed in both breasts?

➤ Has there been breast cancer in more than one generation of your family?

➤ Are you of Eastern or Central European Jewish heritage?

Other factors that appear to increase your risk for breast cancer include being obese, being age 30 or older at the birth of your first child or never having been pregnant, indulging in heavy alcohol consumption, and eating a high-fat diet.

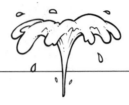

### Wellspring

In 1994, researchers discovered that hereditary defects in two genes can increase a woman's risk for developing breast cancer. Called BRCA1 and BRCA2, these genes normally play a role in cell repair functions. If defective, however, these genes can instead spur the growth of cancer cells in breast tissue. Researchers believe that BRCA1 and BRCA2 defects are responsible for 95 percent of all inherited forms of breast cancer (which account for only 5 percent of breast cancers overall). Although the average woman has a greater than 90 percent chance of never developing breast cancer during her lifetime, a woman with a BRCA1 or BRCA2 defect has up to a 90 percent chance of getting breast cancer by age 85.

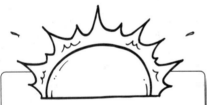

### Embracing Change

Some women at high risk for breast cancer can lower their risk by taking the drug tamoxifen after menopause, which is a selective estrogen receptor moderator (SERM). Tamoxifen appears to block estrogen from reaching breast tissue, thwarting the development of breast cancer. This doesn't prevent cancer entirely, but it does cut in half the risk that it will develop.

## HRT and Breast Cancer

There is concern about the relationship between HRT and breast cancer. Breast cancer is often hormone-driven, which means that it thrives on estrogen. In addition, some studies indicate that the progesterone added to HRT to reduce the risk for endometrial cancer could also increase the risk for breast cancer. There seems to be no change in cancer risk for the first five years that you take HRT, which is good news if you've been taking HRT primarily to manage the discomforts of menopause. However, taking HRT for longer than 10 years appears to increase your risk of developing breast cancer by about a third.

Before you panic and throw the rest of your HRT prescription down the toilet, remember that risk is relative. If you have no other risk factors for breast cancer, long-term HRT use may change your risk from 1 in 12 to 1 in 9. If you have other risk factors, such as being overweight, HRT could increase your breast cancer risk to 1 in 7 or greater. Breast cancer risk is only one of many factors to consider when evaluating HRT, however. If you're worried about breast cancer because you're taking HRT, talk with your doctor about your overall health risks.

## *What You Can Do to Help Keep Your Breasts Healthy*

BSE is the most important thing that you can do for your breast health. You know your breasts better than anyone else can, and you are the best one to know if they change. After age 40, you should also have annual clinical breast exams, or CBEs, from your gynecologist or women's healthcare provider. If your doctor recommends, or you want to have, annual mammograms, that's another way to monitor your breast health. Healthy lifestyle habits such as eating a low-fat diet, exercising regularly, increasing your intake of soy, and limiting alcohol consumption can also help.

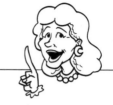

**Wise Woman's Wisdom**

"I am not afraid of storms for I am learning how to sail my ship."

—Louisa May Alcott

# Creating Healthy Self-Care Habits

Knowledge is your most important asset when it comes to safeguarding your health after menopause. The better you know your body, the more easily you can detect changes with potentially harmful consequences. Because there appear to be links between certain cancers and a high-fat diet, and between a lower cancer risk overall and regular exercise, pay attention to these lifestyle factors. Of course, you can't prevent every health problem. But you can minimize the likelihood that health problems will interfere with the quality and length of your life.

### The Least You Need to Know

➤ The human papilloma virus (HPV), which causes genital warts, also causes nearly all cases of cervical cancer. Preventing HPV infection could eliminate your risk for cervical cancer.

➤ The most important thing you can do for breast health is to do regular BSEs. BSE detects more cancers in their early stages than any other assessment method.

➤ Women who are at high risk for hereditary breast cancer should discuss ways to lower their risks, such as taking tamoxifen, with their gynecologists.

➤ Although mammograms can produce false-positive findings, they can also detect cancer before the tumor is big enough for you or your doctor to feel.

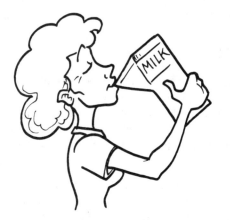

# Chapter 27

# Staying Healthy After Menopause: Inner Changes

## In This Chapter

➤ Why your bones lose calcium after menopause

➤ How to prevent and treat osteoporosis

➤ How HRT affects osteoporosis

➤ What happens to your heart after menopause

➤ How HRT affects heart disease

➤ How to keep your mind sharp and alert

On the outside, you look strong and healthy. Is that a reflection of what's on the in-side? In many cases, yes. Vibrant skin and firm muscles reflect a body that's getting good nutrition and regular physical activity. It's limber and flexible, able to leap tall buildings in a single bound—oh, wait, wrong superhero. This is the woman who sel-dom looks or acts her age, able to run with the wolves (urban or wild).

In some circumstances, however, looks are deceiving. Menopause causes endless changes in your body. Your lower estrogen level affects the way your body metabolizes lipids and fatty acids, for example, which often results in higher blood cholesterol lev-els that can lead to coronary artery disease. That fit and trim body, if it belongs to a woman of slight build, could hide bones as fragile as porcelain.

In Chapter 26, "Staying Healthy After Menopause: Outer Changes," we discussed the obvious changes that take place in your body. This chapter discusses the changes you can't see and the health consequences they can have.

# Building Strength for Maturity

Your body is capable of great strength at any age. It's just that the older you are, the more it takes to develop that strength—and the quicker it disappears in the face of challenge. By the time you're in your 40s and 50s, your body's ability to extract nutrients from the foods you eat is beginning to diminish. Your body works harder and gets less for its efforts. This reduces the building materials available to your body to replace cells and repair tissues.

And in case you haven't yet noticed, fat tissue is beginning to replace muscle tissue throughout your body, a consequence of lower estrogen levels. The same workout that gave you pleasantly firm and defined muscles when you were in your 30s won't have quite the same effect now, because your body has less muscle tissue to work out. Your lower estrogen levels also reduce the elasticity of your body's connective tissues, making your joints less flexible and increasing your risk for injury. Arthritis, an inflammation of the connective tissues around your joints, might also cause stiffening and even pain with strenuous movements.

The good news is that your efforts to strengthen and condition your body will have positive and far-reaching results. Regular movement is the most effective means of maintaining flexibility even in the presence of conditions such as arthritis. Your muscles will grow strong, improving your balance and reducing your risk for injury. And most importantly, regular exercise strengthens your bones.

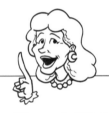

**Wise Woman's Wisdom**

"True strength is delicate."

—Louise Nevelson

## *Osteoporosis: Preventing Brittle Bones*

Although we think of bones as solid structures, they're actually hollow and made mostly of water. What gives them their solid form is calcium—specifically, calcium phosphate in combination with collagen, a form of protein that provides a framework that the calcium phosphate causes to harden.

For all your life, your bones exist in a state of give and take. Your body reabsorbs old bone tissue that's worn out and replaces it with new bone tissue that's fresh and strong. From birth until about age 25 or so, your body gives more than it takes, building more new bone than reabsorbing old bone. Your skeleton continues to grow until it reaches peak bone mass sometime during your mid-20s. By age 30, the balance shifts and your body starts to take more than it gives. It continues to build new bone tissue, but at a much slower pace. Reabsorption usually continues at the same rate, although it can sometimes accelerate.

Losing estrogen at menopause causes the "give" part of the formula to slow even more. In the first five to seven years after menopause, you can end up with a net loss of 20 percent of your bone mass just as a consequence of the changes of menopause. The imbalance can also accelerate the reabsorption process, further diminishing bone density.

*Osteoporosis* is a condition that occurs when your bone density slips below a certain threshold—typically a 15 to 20 percent loss. Although we used to call this "brittle bone disease," we now know that the problem is not one of brittleness, but of porousness. The loss of calcium leaves bone tissue looking somewhat lacelike. In this state, the bone lacks structural strength. It's quite fragile and fractures easily, sometimes spontaneously (with no apparent cause).

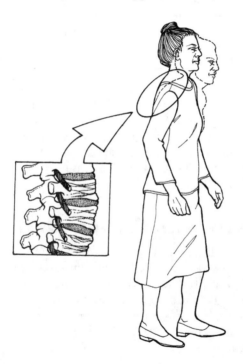

*Work to prevent the effects of osteoporosis by supplementing your diet with calcium and increasing your strength through a personalized fitness program that includes weight-bearing exercise. Talk to your doctor about it.*

## Bone Density Testing

Bone density testing measures the mineral content of your bones. One of the most accurate procedures is called dual energy x-ray absorptiometry, or DEXA. DEXA takes a special x-ray of your spine or your hip that shows demineralization—the loss of calcium and other essential minerals that give your bones strength and stability. DEXA is rather expensive and isn't always covered by health insurance. Some clinics now

### Wise Up

**Osteoporosis** is a disease in which your bones experience so much mineral loss, particularly calcium, that they appear porous and spongelike. The word *osteoporosis* means "porous bone."

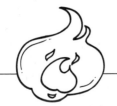

### Hot Flash!

Are you shrinking? Although it's normal for everyone's height to decrease as a normal aspect of aging (the disks in your spine compress), a height loss of more than 1 inch could signal abnormal bone loss and osteoporosis.

have portable DEXA machines that measure the density of a bone in your finger or heel. These are less expensive but somewhat less accurate, although they still give a good overview of your bone density status. DEXA can reveal mineral loss of less than 10 percent. By contrast, conventional x-rays can show calcium loss after it reaches about 25 percent, generally a point at which fractures are occurring.

Another form of bone density testing uses an ultrasound reading done on your heel. This test sends sound waves painlessly through your heel. The denser the bone, the longer it takes the sound waves to go through. Unlike the ultrasound that shows images of internal body parts such as your heart or ovaries, bone density ultrasound reports its measurements in numbers that your doctor then interprets.

The American Osteoporosis Foundation recommends that women age 65 and older have a bone density test every year. You should have a bone density test if you're under age 65 if you have additional risk factors for osteoporosis. Such risk factors include a slight build, menopause before age 45, recent fractures, hyperthyroidism or type 1 diabetes, or steroids taken to treat chronic inflammatory diseases such as asthma or rheumatoid arthritis.

## Calcium In, Calcium Out

Calcium is a crucial element when it comes to preventing osteoporosis. The calcium intake that matters most, unfortunately, takes place before age 25, when your body is still building more bone than it's reclaiming. The greater your bone density when your bone mass peaks, the less likely you are to develop osteoporosis.

After about age 50, your body metabolizes nutrients, including calcium, less efficiently. Yet calcium is a vital element—your body needs it for cell repair and to maintain the electrical circuitry that keeps your heart beating. If there's not enough calcium in your bloodstream to supply your body's needs, then your body makes a withdrawal from the First Personal Bank of Calcium: your bones. This further reduces the mineral content of your bones, decreasing their density.

Most women benefit from taking calcium supplements. It's often difficult to reach the recommended intake of 1,500 mg a day through diet alone. And there's some evidence that your body more readily absorbs calcium in certain supplemental forms. Although the effect is weaker than that of estrogen, calcium supplements appear to slow bone reabsorption. Calcium supplements are most effective for women who have normal bone density and want to keep it that way. Women who already have significant bone loss need additional treatment.

Calcium supplements can be confusing because calcium doesn't come by itself. It's not stable alone, so it's always blended with another chemical. The most common combinations are calcium carbonate, calcium citrate, calcium lactate, and calcium gluconate. The elemental calcium—"raw" calcium—that each of these products contains varies. Calcium carbonate contains the highest percentage of elemental calcium (40 percent), although some health experts believe that your body more easily absorbs calcium citrate (21 percent elemental calcium). Calcium carbonate is also the least expensive calcium supplement and is the main ingredient in products such as TUMS.

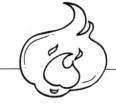

**Hot Flash!**

Calcium supplements made from bone meal or dolomite (oyster shells) may contain toxic substances such as lead, mercury, and arsenic. Look for brands with "USP" on the label. These manufacturers have agreed to the standards set by the U.S. Pharmacopoeia for quality and purity.

Magnesium and vitamin D are just as important as calcium when it comes to safeguarding the health of your bones. These substances are necessary for your body to absorb and use calcium. Many supplement preparations include calcium, magnesium, and vitamin D to assure that you get adequate levels of all three.

## Elemental Calcium Content of Common Calcium Supplements

| Supplement | Percent of Elemental Calcium | Amount of Supplement Needed to Provide 200 mg of Elemental Calcium |
| --- | --- | --- |
| Calcium carbonate | 40 percent | 500 mg |
| Calcium citrate | 21 percent | 950 mg |
| Calcium lactate | 13 percent | 1,500 mg |
| Calcium gluconate | 9 percent | 2,200 mg |

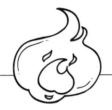

**Hot Flash!**

Back off the colas to save your bones. Cola and root beer soft drinks contain phosphoric acid, which acts like a magnet to draw calcium from your bones. If you absolutely must drink soda, choose something that's clear (and sugar–free).

## Gaining Strength Through Weight-Bearing Exercise

A funny thing can happen on your walks around the block: You can close the First Personal Bank of Calcium, or at least some of its branches. Weight-bearing exercise such as walking or jogging slows the loss of calcium from the bones that the activity affects—most often your legs, hips, and lower spine. Weight resistance training can have the same effect on your upper body, strengthening the bones in your arms and upper back. Regular exercise has the added value of improving your balance and coordination. This reduces your risk of falling, which is the leading cause of fractures.

## Treatments from the Pharmacy

Unfortunately, there are as yet no treatments that cause your body to develop new bone tissue. All treatment efforts focus on halting the loss of additional bone tissue and supplying enough calcium to strengthen the bone tissue that remains. Estrogen does this the most effectively, making HRT the leading treatment to prevent osteoporosis. Other medications target specific aspects of osteoporosis. These are some of the more common ones:

➤ **Alendronate**, which belongs to the group of drugs called bisphosphonates, is particularly effective for women taking medications such as steroids that cause bone density loss. Alendronate (common brand name Fosamax) slows bone re-absorption and increases bone density in the spine and hips.

➤ **Raloxifene** (common brand name Evista) belongs to a class of drugs called selective estrogen receptor modulators (SERMs). It provides some estrogenlike benefits, such as reduced bone loss, without some of the risks (such as increased risk for breast cancer).

➤ **Calcitonin** is a naturally occurring hormone that plays a key role in calcium metabolism. It is most effective in women who are at least five years beyond menopause by slowing the loss of bone tissue and improving bone density in the spine.

## Therapies from Nature

Foods naturally high in calcium help your body get the dietary calcium that it needs to build new bone tissue and to meet its other needs for calcium, which reduces calcium withdrawal from your bones. Foods that are good sources of dietary calcium include low-fat dairy products and green, leafy vegetables such as spinach.

Phytoestrogens, such as those found in soy and red clover supplements, may also be effective in reducing bone loss. Although they're weaker than estrogen replacements, phytoestrogens act in similar ways in your body. Researchers are still exploring whether the effect is strong enough to help in moderate to severe cases of osteoporosis. At this point, most health experts believe that women who show signs of osteoporosis should consider stronger treatments.

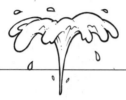

### Wellspring

Recent research suggests that drugs commonly prescribed to lower blood cholesterol levels, called statins, also stimulate the growth of new bone tissue. This is significant for two reasons. First, statins have been in use for about 20 years and have few side effects. Second, this is the first product to cause new bone tissue to grow. Other drugs to treat osteoporosis work by preventing further loss of bone, not by encouraging new bone growth. They also have significant risks and side effects, including an increased risk for certain cancers. More research is still needed to determine who will benefit most from statins and whether statins can sustain bone growth over the long term.

## Bone Density and Breast Cancer

Ironically, there is a relationship between higher bone density and its related lower risk of osteoporosis and a higher risk for breast cancer. The link again appears to be estrogen. Higher estrogen levels keep your bones stronger. But higher estrogen levels also increase your risk for breast cancer. Is it a worthwhile trade-off? It depends on your individual health circumstances. Osteoporosis causes nearly two million fractures a year, many of which result in lasting disability. Heart disease is the leading cause of death in America, causing the deaths of one out of every two women—more than all cancers combined.

# The Heart of the Matter

Your heart nestles in the center of your chest, safe behind the bony armor of your ribs and sternum, steadily beating out the rhythm of your life. It contracts and

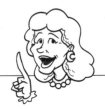

**Wise Woman's Wisdom**

"Talk happiness: talk faith: talk health. Say you are well, or all is well with you, and God shall hear your words and make them true."

—Ella Wheeler-Wilcox

expands 100,000 times a day, sending blood coursing through your body at a rate equal to 75 gallons an hour. The network of arteries, veins, and capillaries that sends this blood to every cell in your body would, if lined up end to end, cover nearly 100,000 miles.

Pretty impressive, but what does this have to do with menopause? Well, all that estrogen that flows through your body before menopause helps keep your heart and blood vessels in prime operating condition. When menopause cuts that flow back to nearly nothing, your cardiac system responds by becoming more like a man's. This doesn't mean that your heart gets bigger and stronger. To the contrary, it might actually become flabbier and less efficient.

## Why Your Risk for Heart Disease Increases

As a woman, before menopause your risk for heart disease is significantly less than the risk that a man of the same age and general health status faces. After menopause, your risk begins to increase until, by age 80 or so, it's about the same as a man's. Although doctors suspect that estrogen is a key part of the reason for this, researchers have not yet been able to pin down precisely what role estrogen plays.

One reason that there is still such uncertainty about estrogen's role is that so many factors contribute to heart disease. No one knows yet which factors are the most critical, although family history is in the lead for that dubious distinction at the present. Some health experts believe that heart disease is eventually inevitable, one of the ways in which the body wears out as it ages. Most, however, believe that nearly all heart disease is fully preventable through proper diet and regular exercise. Still other experts point out that even though a woman's risk of heart disease increases after menopause, it never exceeds a man's risk (all other health factors being equal), whether or not she takes HRT.

## HRT and Heart Disease: The HERS Study

Even research studies about the correlation between HRT and heart disease yield conflicting and inconsistent findings. In 1998, the National Institutes of Health (NIH) completed a four-year study involving nearly 3,000 women past menopause, called the Heart and Estrogen/Progestin Replacement Study (HERS). The HERS study was the first to directly examine the relationship between HRT and heart disease, and the results surprised researchers as well as doctors: HRT seemed to have no effect on events such as heart attacks in women who already had heart disease. Other studies underway hope to provide a better understanding of this finding, although their results won't start becoming available until 2005.

NIH researchers caution women not to give up on HRT solely for this reason. There are many reasons to take or not take HRT, and the potential for reducing the risk of heart disease is just one of many factors to consider. As we said earlier in this chapter, there are still significant benefits on the osteoporosis front. In addition, you need to consider your risk for certain kinds of cancer and other health problems.

## Red Alert: Warning Signs of Heart Trouble

Would you know if you were having a heart attack? You might if your signs were classic: crushing chest pain, breathlessness, and arms so heavy you can't move them. But the reality is, more than half of women (and a third of men) who have heart attacks don't experience any of the traditional symptoms. So, they think it's something else, such as indigestion, the flu, too much stress, or even not enough sleep. But they're wrong—and often, sadly, dead wrong. Studies show that a woman is more likely than a man to die in the critical few weeks following a heart attack.

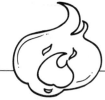

### Hot Flash!

If you think that you could be having a heart attack, don't wait for the "right" symptoms to hit you. Pay attention to your inner wisdom. Seek medical attention immediately. If it's a false alarm, so what? It's better to have family and friends tease you than grieve at your funeral.

## What You Can Do to Keep Your Heart Healthy

Regular exercise and a low-fat diet are the most effective lifestyle choices that you can make to protect the health of your heart. Exercise helps reduce your blood cholesterol levels, lower your blood pressure, and improve the elasticity of your blood vessels. It also tones and conditions the muscle that matters most: your heart.

## Keep This in Mind

Those lower estrogen levels have had an effect in your brain, too. Estrogen appears to enhance the functions of certain neurotransmitters, the biochemicals that help messages travel from one neuron (nerve cell) to another. Researchers believe that the permanent loss of estrogen—for example, when you choose not to take HRT—causes subtle but significant changes in this transmission process. These changes may contribute to memory and cognitive losses, and also to conditions such as Alzheimer's disease. Chapter 10, "A Shift from Left Brain to Right Brain," discusses the correlation between estrogen and functions of the brain.

## Staying Mentally Alert

Like your body, your mind requires regular exercise to keep it in prime working order. Because midlife can be a time when activities that stretch your thinking and reasoning abilities are starting to diminish—for example, if you retire from your job or shift to working just part-time—it's important to be sure that you keep your brain busy. If your work is less mentally challenging these days, fill the gap with other activities such as reading. Research shows that older people who play musical instruments, play organized games such as cards or chess, and do crossword puzzles stimulate the parts of their brains responsible for thought and analysis far more extensively than people who pass the time watching television.

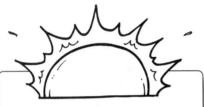

**Embracing Change**

For more information about heart health, see *The Complete Idiot's Guide to a Happy Healthy Heart,* by Deborah S. Romaine and Dawn E. DeWitt, M.D. (Alpha Books, 1998).

## HRT and Alzheimer's Disease

Researchers don't fully understand the relationship between estrogen and Alzheimer's disease, although they know that one exists. Women who take HRT following menopause have a lower risk for developing Alzheimer's disease than women who choose not to take HRT. Doctors believe that at least part of the explanation lies in the ability of estrogen to stimulate neurotransmitters called acetycholines. These substances directly participate in storing and retrieving memories. One theory is that estrogen is like a lubricant that keeps the acetycholines from becoming entangled. When estrogen levels drop, this effect decreases. HRT, of course, boosts estrogen levels back up again.

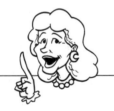

**Wise Woman's Wisdom**

"When you trust your intuition, you get more of the truth—and you get it faster than using your intellect."

—Barbara Braham

## The Wise Woman's Wisdom

Do you find that you are more willing to accept a "gut" response about a situation? After menopause, the barriers between intellect and intuition seem to crumble. Your women's intuition comes into full bloom. It's not that you've abandoned your critical thinking skills. Instead, you've expanded them. What you've abandoned are your attempts to be in conscious control of your thought processes. You allow yourself to respond without interfering, letting answers just come to you.

This ability can serve you well when it comes to matters of your health. Often you'll just have a vague feeling that something's not right. Check it out. Even if it turns out to be a minor problem, it's a message from your body. Many women schedule appointments with their doctors for seemingly minor matters and then discover a more serious potential problem lurking in the shadows. When your body speaks to you, listen. You're connected now, like you've never been connected before.

# The Heart and Soul of a Healthy Body-Mind

How you feel about life beyond menopause has a great influence on how events unfold. Although it may sound trite to say that a positive attitude can carry you a long way, there's much truth in the words. Doctors have long known, for example, that a positive attitude can make the difference in coming through a life-threatening situation such as cancer. You can't will good health, of course. But you can provide the mind-set that encourages you to find the best in whatever state of health you find yourself.

---

### The Least You Need to Know

➤ Lower estrogen levels after menopause increase your risk for osteoporosis and heart disease.

➤ Regular exercise and good nutrition can delay and possibly prevent both osteoporosis and heart disease.

➤ It's crucial to get enough calcium in your daily diet, either through the foods that you eat, calcium supplements, or a combination of both.

➤ Researchers don't yet know whether phytoestrogens provide the same benefits as HRT when it comes to osteoporosis and heart disease.

➤ Intuition is a sign that your body and mind are communicating. It's up to you to pay attention.

---

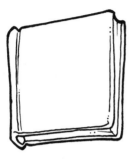

# Glossary

**abdominal hysterectomy**   Surgery to remove the uterus through an incision in the abdomen.

**abnormal uterine bleeding (AUB)**   Vaginal bleeding that is irregular, heavy, and unusual, and that may be a sign of potentially serious health problems.

**acupuncture**   Ancient Chinese therapy that uses hairlike needles inserted into certain locations along the body's energy pathways.

**allopathic medicine**   Conventional Western medicine practiced by M.D.s (medical doctors) and often in the United States by D.O.s (doctors of osteopathy).

**Alzheimer's disease**   A progressive, incurable condition in which the nerve cells in the brain degenerate, resulting in loss of cognitive (thinking) ability and memory.

**androgens**   The hormones responsible for secondary sex characteristics in men and libido in both genders.

**antioxidant**   A substance that binds with the byproducts of metabolism (called free radicals) to keep them from becoming poisons within the body.

**aphrodisiac**   Substance believed to improve sex drive.

**assisted reproductive technology (ART)**   A group of high-tech procedures that produce conception without sexual intercourse.

**autoimmune disorder**   A health condition in which your body produces substances that attack its own tissues or organs.

**ayurveda**   The traditional medicine of India, which has been practiced for more than 5,000 years.

**bioequivalent**   A substance that precisely matches the molecular and chemical structure of a substance found naturally in your body.

**biofeedback**   A learned method of consciously altering physical functions that typically take place without conscious effort.

**biopsy**   A small sample of suspicious tissue that is removed and sent to a laboratory for analysis.

**body mass index (BMI)**   A mathematical calculation that categorizes a person's risk for health problems as it relates to body weight.

**bone density**   The amount of minerals, especially calcium, contained in bones.

**botanical**   A plant-based substance or product used for therapeutic or healing purposes.

**breast self-exam (BSE)**   A technique for systematically exploring your own breasts to detect unusual lumps.

**cerebrum**   The largest and most developed of the three physical parts of the human brain that handles all conscious and mental processes, including thought and memory.

**chakras**   The centers of energy within your body.

**chi**   The life energy that supports your existence.

**cholesterol**   A specific family of lipoproteins, made naturally in the human body and found in red meats and dairy products, that are used to make cell membranes and manufacture hormones.

**climacteric**   A word sometimes used to refer to menopause that means significant turning point or critical phase in a sequence of events.

**complementary therapies**   Any healing approaches that are outside the realm of allopathic medicine.

**conjugated estrogens**   A form of HRT that contains two or more different forms of estrogen in combination.

**coumestans**   The phytoestrogens found in legumes (also called coumesterols).

**daily values (DVs)**   The amounts and percentages of nutrients that packaged foods contain, based on FDA-established minimum nutritional requirements for healthy adults.

**doctrine of humors**   An ancient model of medicine based on the link between vital body fluids and the elements that those fluids represented; it formed the core of Eastern and Western medical practices for thousands of years.

**dysfunctional uterine bleeding (DUB)**   Moderate, predictable bleeding that occurs as the body's hormone levels fluctuate; it is not usually a sign of any health problems.

**early menopause**   Menopause that occurs when a woman is in her early 40s or younger.

**elective surgery**   Surgery that is necessary but not urgent.

**endocrine system**   The network of the body's glands and hormones.

**endorphins**   The morphinelike chemicals that the brain naturally produces to relieve pain.

**estrogen**   The collective name for the group of hormones responsible for a woman's secondary sexual characteristics and many functions of the reproductive cycle.

**estrogen receptors**   The protein molecules within the body's tissue cells that connect to the molecules in estrogens.

**fibroid**   An abnormal growth of muscle and connective tissue that forms in the uterus.

**FSH**   Follicle-stimulating hormone.

**glands**   The structures within the body that produce hormones.

**herbalist**   A person specially trained in using herbs and other botanicals for therapeutic purposes.

**homeopathy**   A system of medicine that uses tiny amounts of natural substances to stimulate the body's own healing mechanisms.

**hormone replacement therapy (HRT)**   Prescription drugs taken to restore levels of some of the hormones that naturally diminish during and after menopause.

**hormones**   The chemical messengers that the body produces that stimulate or initiate certain events or actions inside the body.

**hypothyroidism**   A medical condition in which the thyroid gland fails to produce adequate levels of thyroxin and other hormones.

**hysterectomy**   The surgical removal of the uterus. May be abdominal or vaginal.

**hysteroscopy**   A procedure during which the doctor passes a flexible, lighted, magnifying scope through the vagina and cervix into the uterus to look for abnormalities.

**infertility**   The situation of being unable to conceive.

**insulin-dependent diabetes**   A medical condition in which the pancreas stops producing the hormone insulin.

**integrative medicine**   A therapeutic approach that seeks to blend and balance various methods to provide a holistic or unified approach to wellness as well as treatment.

**iron-deficiency anemia**   A health condition in which the blood's red cells are low in hemoglobin, reducing their ability to carry oxygen.

**isoflavones**   The group of phytoestrogens found in soy.

**journaling**   The process of using writing to explore your thoughts and ideas.

**kundalini**   The most powerful of the energies contained in the chakras that resides within the root, or first, chakra.

**laparoscopic hysterectomy**   A hysterectomy, leaving the cervix behind, that is performed by inserting instruments through several small incisions in the abdomen.

**laparoscopically assisted vaginal hysterectomy (LAVH)**   A hysterectomy performed by inserting special lighted instruments through small incisions in the abdomen to remove the uterus and sometimes also the fallopian tubes and ovaries.

**labyrinth**   A single, or unicursal, path that follows a number of circuits before ending up in the center.

**left brain**   The part of the brain responsible for linear thought and functions such as logic and analysis.

**legumes**   Plants that produce fruits or seeds (such as beans or peas) that humans can eat.

**libido**   A person's sex drive or interest in sexual activity.

**lignans**   A group of phytoestrogens.

**lipoproteins**   The fatty acids within the body.

**low-dose birth control pills**   Oral contraceptive pills that contain lower doses of hormones than standard birth control pills; sometimes used to support fluctuating hormone levels during perimenopause.

**mammogram**   An x-ray of the breasts.

**melatonin**   A natural hormone the body produces that causes sleepiness.

**menopause**   The ending of a woman's monthly menstrual periods.

**metaphysical**   A term that means "beyond or around the physical" and that typically describes experiences that involve the body, mind, and spirit as a collective whole.

**monophasic birth control pills**   Oral contraceptive pills that contain the same levels of estrogen and progesterone in each active pill, unlike other birth control pills that contain varying levels of hormones for different weeks of the menstrual cycle.

**nadis**   The unseen pathways that connect the chakras.

**naturopathy**   A system of healing that uses remedies found in nature, such as plants and herbs.

**neuropeptides**   The amino acids that convey messages between the brain and the body.

**organic produce**   Fruits and vegetables that are planted, cultivated, harvested, and stored without any chemical additives such as fertilizers, insecticides, herbicides, and preservatives.

**osteopathy**   A system of medicine that views the body as a unified structure with the musculoskeletal system as its core.

**osteoporosis**   A potentially serious health condition in which the bones lose calcium, becoming fragile and susceptible to fractures.

**Pap test**   A laboratory test that detects cancerous cells scraped from the surface of the cervix.

**peer review**   A formal process through which professionals of comparable expertise assess a study's methods and structures for reliability and scientific soundness.

**perimenopause**   The period of time, usually ranging from two to six years, when a woman's body is preparing for menopause.

**phenolic estrogens**   The chemical family to which phytoestrogens belong.

**phytoestrogens**   The substances found in certain plants and seeds that are chemically similar to estrogen.

**polycystic ovary syndrome (PCOS)**   A metabolic condition in which the ovaries develop numerous cysts that interfere with follicle function and egg production.

**polyp**   An abnormal growth that can form in mucous membrane tissue such as the cervix.

**premature menopause**   A form of early menopause that occurs when a woman is in her 20s or 30s.

**premature ovarian failure**   A condition in which the ovaries stop functioning well ahead of the normal time of menopause, without obvious precipitating medical conditions or surgery.

**premenstrual syndrome (PMS)**   A collection of symptoms that begin after ovulation and usually conclude when menstruation starts.

**primary amenorrhea**   A condition in which a young woman's menstrual periods never start, without the presence of any medical conditions that could cause amenorrhea (absence of menstruation).

**progesterone**   A hormone produced in the corpus luteum cyst on the ovary that is involved in the female reproductive cycle that stimulates the thickening of the uterus wall in preparation for pregnancy.

**radical hysterectomy**   Surgical removal of the uterus, the cervix, the upper portion of the vagina, both ovaries and fallopian tubes, and surrounding lymph glands, typically as a treatment for cervical cancer.

**Reiki**   A Japanese healing method in which the practitioner uses her hands to focus energy over afflicted body parts.

**317**

**resorcyclic acid lactones**   The phytoestrogens that occur in grains such as rice, corn, barley, and wheat.

**right brain**   The part of the brain responsible for nonlinear thought and creativity.

**selective estrogen receptor modulators (SERMs)**   A group of drugs that produce some, but not all, effects of estrogen.

**serotonin**   A natural substance in the brain that is related to feelings of well-being, as well as depression.

**steroidal estrogens**   The estrogens that the body produces.

**subfertility**   The natural reduction in fertility that occurs as a result of aging.

**subtotal hysterectomy**   Surgery to remove just the uterus, leaving behind the cervix.

**testosterone**   A hormone responsible for secondary sexual characteristics in men and sex drive in women.

**thermoregulatory dysfunction**   The technical term for the hot flashes and chills that often occur during menopause.

**total hysterectomy**   Surgery to remove the uterus and the cervix.

**total hysterectomy with bilateral salpingo-oophorectomy**   Surgery to remove the uterus, cervix, fallopian tubes, and ovaries.

**traditional Chinese medicine (TCM)**   An ancient form of medicine that incorporates acupuncture and herbal remedies.

**transdermal patch**   A method for taking HRT that transmits the drug through the skin and directly into the bloodstream.

**vaginal hysterectomy**   The least invasive surgery for removing the uterus, in which the surgeon works through an incision inside the vagina at the top along the cervix.

**vasomotor regulation**   The process by which the body maintains a stable temperature.

**weight-bearing exercise**   Moderate to intense physical activity, such as jogging or walking, that puts pressure on your skeletal system.

**yang**   A form of energy that represents the warm, light, dry, active, and masculine.

**yin**   A form of energy that represents the cool, dark, moist, passive, and feminine.

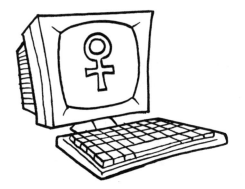

# Resources

There are many resources available if you'd like more information about menopause and related topics. This section identifies books, Web sites, and organizations to help you broaden your knowledge.

## Books

We mention some of these titles in the text of *The Complete Idiot's Guide to Menopause,* but we include others here that provide accurate and insightful information.

Aronson, Diane, and the staff of Resolve. *Resolving Infertility* (HarperCollins, 1999).

Budilovsky, Joan, and Eve Adamson. *The Complete Idiot's Guide to Meditation* (Alpha Books, 1998).

———. *The Complete Idiot's Guide to Yoga* (Alpha Books, 1998).

Cabot, Sandra, M.D. *Smart Medicine for Menopause* (Avery Publication Group, 1998).

Canfield, Jack, and Mark Victor Hansen. *The Aladdin Factor* (Berkeley Books, 1995).

Carper, Jean. *Food—Your Miracle Medicine* (HarperCollins, 1993).

Domar, Alice, Ph.D., and Dreher, Henry. *Healing Mind, Healthy Woman* (Delta, 1997).

Gittleman, Ann Louise, M.S., C.N.S. *Before the Change: Taking Charge of Your Perimenopause* (Harper San Francisco, 1999).

Gottlieb, Bill, ed. *New Choices in Natural Healing* (Rodale Press, 1995).

Lark, Susan M., M.D. *Women's Health Companion: A Self-Help Nutrition Guide and Cookbook* (Celestial Arts, 1996).

Laux, Marcus, N.D., and Conrad, Christine. *Natural Woman, Natural Menopause* (HarperCollins, 1998).

Lee, John R., M.D., and Hopkins, Virginia. *What Your Doctor May Not Tell You About Menopause* (Warner Books, 1996).

Love, Susan, M.D. *Dr. Susan Love's Hormone Book: Making Informed Choices About Menopause* (Random House, 1998).

Magee, Elaine. *Eat Well for a Healthy Menopause* (John Wiley & Sons, 1997).

Nelson, Miriam E., Ph.D., with Wernick, Sarah, Ph.D. *Strong Women Stay Young: Revised Edition* (Bantam Doubleday Dell, 2000).

Northrup, Christiane, M.D. *Women's Bodies, Women's Wisdom: Creating Physical and Emotional Health and Healing* (Bantam Doubleday Dell, 1998).

Romaine, Deborah S., and Dawn E. DeWitt, M.D. *The Complete Idiot's Guide to a Happy Healthy Heart* (Alpha Books, 1998).

Rosenthal, Saul H., M.D., and Jeremy P. Tarcher. *The New Sex Over 40* (Putnam, 1999).

Shandler, Nina. *Estrogen the Natural Way* (Villard Books, 1998).

Zand, Janet, LAc, OMD, Spreen, Allan N., M.D., C.N.C., and LaValle, James B., R.Ph., N.D. *Smart Medicine for Healthier Living* (Avery Publishing Group, 1999).

# Organizations

**National Institute on Aging (NIA)**
Building 31, Room 5C27
31 Center Drive, MSC 2292
Bethesda, MD 20892
Phone: 301-496-1752
Web site: www.nih.gov/nia/

The NIA provides a broad range of information about topics related to aging, including health and wellness, sexuality, demographics, and various statistics.

**National Institutes of Health Osteoporosis and Related Bone Diseases—National Resource Center (ORBD-NRC)**
1232 22nd Street NW
Washington, D.C.
Phone: 1-800-624-2663
Web site: www.osteo.org

The ORBD-NRC provides fact sheets, news articles, and research information about osteoporosis and related bone conditions. The National Osteoporosis Foundation operates the Web site for the ORBD-NRC.

**National Osteoporosis Foundation**
1232 22nd Street NW
Washington, D.C.
Phone: 202-223-2226
Web site: www.nof.org

The National Osteoporosis Foundation sponsors and reports on research on osteoporosis. The organization also supports education and awareness programs that target people at risk for developing osteoporosis.

**American Cancer Society (ACS)**
Phone: 1-800-227-2345
Web site: www.cancer.org

The ACS works to eliminate cancer as a health risk through education, prevention, early detection, and effective treatment. The organization also supports research, advocacy, and public policy to find new treatments and cures, and provides free health education materials for consumers and healthcare professionals. The American Cancer Society operates from local and regional locations listed in your telephone directory.

**American Heart Association (AHA)**
National Center
7272 Greenville Avenue
Dallas, TX 75231
Women's Health Information Phone: 1-888-694-3278
Web site: www.amhrt.org

The American Heart Association provides extensive educational information and materials about all aspects of heart disease, including a special focus on women's health issues. The AHA sponsors the online women's heart health program called "Choose to Move" (www.justmove.org).

**The North American Menopause Society (NAMS)**
P.O. Box 94527
Cleveland, OH 44101-4527
Phone: 440-442-7550
Web site: www.menopause.org

The NAMS is a not-for-profit scientific organization devoted to promoting understanding of menopause and women's health at midlife and beyond. The Web site provides information for consumers as well as healthcare professionals.

# Web Sites

**www.families-first.com/hotflash/**

This is a jazzy commercial site with current information about menopause and related topics, including books for sale and a masthead of experts who answer questions and provide suggestions. The site also sponsors online support groups.

**www.menopauseonline.com**

This Web site provides information about integrative approaches to treating the discomforts and potential health concerns of menopause. There are in-depth articles about holistic, as well as allopathic, therapies.

**www.onhealth.com**

This Web site is an excellent source for information about complementary, as well as conventional (allopathic), therapies.

**www.pofsupport.org**

This is the Web site for the Premature Ovarian Failure support group. It features articles, research findings, membership information, local support groups, and links to related sites.

**www.resolve.org**

This is the Web site for Resolve, the national infertility association. The mission of Resolve is to provide timely, compassionate support and information to people who are experiencing infertility. Resolve has a network of local chapters nationwide, and features national and chapter HelpLines, e-mail service, and fact sheets and publications. Resolve is an excellent resource for women and couples over 40 who want to have a baby at midlife.

**www.wholehealthMD.com**

This Web site provides comprehensive and balanced information about complementary therapies and integrative medicine. It features an extensive index of herbal remedies.

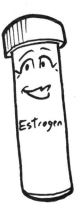

# Hormones at a Glance

Lowering levels of these key hormones cause menopause to occur.

| Hormone | Produced by | Functions | Effects of Loss |
|---|---|---|---|
| Estrogen (estradiol) | Ovaries, fat cells | Causes eggs to mature, affects lipids, affects bone development, affects memory and cognition | Causes end of periods, hot flashes, mood swings, PMS-like symptoms, vaginal dryness, memory and thought disturbances; can elevate blood lipid levels; accelerates mineral loss from bones |
| Follicle-stimulating hormone (FSH) | Pituitary gland | Cause ovaries to increase estrogen output to cause ovulation | Causes elevated FSH levels that remain high after menopause |

*continues*

*continued*

| Hormone | Produced by | Functions | Effects of Loss |
|---|---|---|---|
| Progesterone | Ovaries | Causes uterus lining to thicken to support pregnancy; results in menstruation if no pregnancy occurs | Uterine tissue thins and shrinks |
| Testosterone | Ovaries, adrenal glands | Regulates sex drive; affects energy levels | Possibly reduces sex drive and energy |

# Index

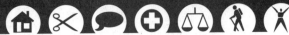
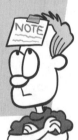